D0892524

Making the most of the time you have

Sarah Christie

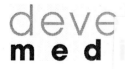

B59921

Published by Developmedica 2009
Castle Court
Duke Street
New Basford,
Nottingham, NG7 7JN
0845 838 0571
www.developmedica.com

The views expressed in this book are those of Developmedica and not those of the National Health Service. Developmedica is in no way associated with the National Health Service.

The contents of this book are intended as a guide only and although every effort has been made to ensure that the contents of this book are correct, Developmedica cannot be held responsible for the outcome of any loss or damage that results from the use of this guide. Readers are advised to seek independent advice regarding their Time Management skills in the workplace.

Every effort has been made to contact the copyright holders of any material reproduced within this publication. If any have been inadvertently overlooked, the publishers will be pleased to make restitution at the earliest opportunity.

A catalogue record for this title is available from the British Library

ISBN 978-1-906839-08-6

Typeset by Replika Press Pvt. Ltd. (India)

Printed by Bell and Bain, Glasgow

1 2 3 4 5 6 7 8 9 10

Contents

About the author

Sarah Christie is a professional performance coach and personal development trainer who specialises in time management. With over 20 years' experience in corporate organisations, Sarah has successfully transitioned theories and techniques from the business world into the medical environment. She has worked as a freelance trainer for Developmedica since 2007. Having worked with doctors for so many years she now considers herself a doctor in spirit and believes she has developed a greater understanding of the pressures doctors face in modern medicine.

Acknowledgements

I would like to thank Matt Green for giving me the opportunity to write this book and my family who have shown great patience and support through the long months it has taken.

In particular I would like to thank my editor, Jen Neal, who has been a constant source of help and encouragement.

Finally, I would like to say a big thank you to the folks who were persuaded by me to read through some chapters and gave their invaluable thoughts and advice.

I appreciate you all!

Foreword – written by a colleague

"The bad news is time flies, the good news is you're the pilot"
– Michael Altshuler

Doctors these days need to have good time management and organisational skills. They have to achieve a blend of lifelong learning and delivering, coupled with work/life balance.

The issue of doctors working long hours is being addressed through government legislation and the European working time directive. However a perfect solution is unlikely. Any change is going to be a slow process with a probably imperfect solution. Consequently doctors will continue to work long hours in the foreseeable future.

Employer demands, patient expectations with low tolerance for mistakes, economic restructuring and the need to keep abreast of medical and technological developments will continue to add to doctors' workload. Therefore, a book on managing priorities is especially required and there has never been a better time for this book.

I have known Sarah for a long time now. She has over 20 years' corporate experience in various management roles, specialising in training, communication and customer service. For the last 3 years she has worked with NHS doctors, delivering programmes in leadership, assertiveness, communication, time management and interviewing skills.

The book itself is well researched, easy to read, and addresses very effectively the issues with time management which most doctors experience. She gives practical strategies to plan and prioritise effectively, and importantly achieve that work/life balance.

Sarah is an educator, and a good one at that. She presents information in a clear and understandable manner. She also wants us to think, and to work! She knows that if you and I want to learn, we have to practise: we have to do the work. Her chapters therefore have exercises. There are skills here that can be acquired, and the format of the book certainly helps.

This book should be of great interest to all, and especially to those who want to excel in their walk of life. Sarah sums it up nicely with Dr. Joseph

Juran's quotation based on the Pareto Principle. We must ask ourselves: do we want to be among the 'vital few or the trivial many?'

I enjoyed the book and found it invaluable. I think you will too. Happy reading!

Mr Uday Dandekar
MS, M.Ch, FRCS (Edin & Glas), FRCSCTh (Edin)
Cardiothoracic Surgeon

Introduction

Time management for busy doctors

Effective time management is a useful skill for anyone in their career, but within medicine it takes on an even greater significance. There are potentially a great many responsibilities and duties that require your time and attention and you may feel yourself pulled in different directions. This can feel chaotic and stressful; therefore, the need for you to take back control of your working day becomes paramount.

About the book

This book aims to offer some insights into the common problems experienced with time management and to provide some techniques and ways of working which can aid greater organisation and productivity. The first three chapters invite you to explore your existing ways of working and to identify the areas that may be undermining your ability to work effectively. The remaining chapters focus on solutions, offering you various techniques to try and improve your current situation. The main theme of the book is about improving the personal effectiveness of clinicians, which means understanding what needs to be done and allocating the time to do it within the clinical day.

The demands of modern medicine

Most doctors recognise only too well the problems of managing their time. Think about all the tasks you have to get done and with whom you need to interact. You have to work with nursing staff, your peers, your supervisors and other health practitioners, all of whom make demands on your working life. You have to interact closely with your patients and their families. You have to organise your time around a long list of clinical duties such as ward rounds, clinics and theatre sessions. You have to continue getting your tasks done even when you are on call which includes not neglecting your administrative tasks such as writing up discharge summaries and dictating notes from your clinics. The clinical environment today requires doctors to undertake teaching sessions, give presentations, attend meetings and sometimes cover for other colleagues' shifts, while continuing with their own development as a doctor. You face many pressures each day with more and more people placing demands on your time. How does that make you feel? Are you able to flourish competently as a doctor? For some who favour a structured day, managing time is easier than it can be for those who do not like to be inhibited by a plan. For most doctors, though, successful time management remains a daunting challenge.

By the time you reach senior levels it is expected that you can manage your working day, understanding that you have to make the most of the resources available, whilst all the time achieving your outcomes, within a constantly changing environment. You need to demonstrate flexibility, decisiveness and be highly organised. You need to identify which activities are going to make you the most productive in the time that you have, remembering you are a role model for your juniors. If you are not a senior doctor yet, but hoping to be, then please ensure you understand what it means to be one within medicine. Time management is relevant to all clinical levels and it will be important to develop these skills now. You are the future leaders and will need to guide others. You will need to focus on what is important, get a strong sense of your priorities and develop an innate determination to get things done. If you do not, you may well be perceived as an ineffectual leader who is not wholly competent. Can you afford to let that happen?

It would be a great disservice to you and your profession if you let such an essential non-clinical skill undermine your undoubted expertise. Take ownership of your personal and professional development. Increase your commitment to improving this skill.

Doctors often take pride in the fact that they work very long hours. However, in modern medicine, this can sometimes be perceived in a negative way. Whether junior or senior, you may run the risk of being considered overwhelmed, unable to cope with your workload and generally not fit for the job. Junior doctors often feel helpless to stand up to senior colleagues but when they stop taking breaks and eating because they 'don't have time', then patient safety may be compromised. There is just too much at stake to ignore time management issues.

The efficiency drivers

There have been two noteworthy events recently which make the need for effective time management non-negotiable for doctors. You will be aware of the introduction of the European Working Time Directive (Working Time Relations, 2003). It came into force in August 2004 to protect the health and safety of doctors in training by reducing hours worked per week to a maximum of 58 and imposing minimum rest requirements with a maximum of 13 hours of work in any 24 and at least 11 hours of rest between shifts. The next challenge has arrived with the full implementation of this directive on the 1st August 2009, which takes the maximum working hours per week down to 48. In early 2009 it was suggested that up to 50% of trusts in the United Kingdom may not be compliant and in some regions this figure was thought to be as low as 30%. The Workforce Review Team analysed 11 broad specialty groups and found that anaesthetics, medicine, obstetrics & gynaecology and surgery had the most doctors working more than 48 hours each week. These specialties all have a high out-of-hours commitment. It is clear that healthcare provision is faced with a big challenge and that significant changes are required to achieve Working Time Directive compliance. In the light of this new standard the need for effective time management has critical implications which cannot be ignored.

The second significant influence on doctors in relation to time management in the United Kingdom is the introduction and implementation of the *Medical Leadership Competency Framework* which has been jointly developed by The Academy of Medical Royal Colleges and the NHS Institute for Innovation and Improvement, in conjunction with a wide range of stakeholders. The *Medical Leadership Competency Framework* applies to all medical students and doctors and is designed to introduce students and doctors at all levels into management and leadership competencies. Although some may not realise it, time management is an important management skill. The ability to be able to organise oneself is the key to eventually being able to organise the activities of whole teams and to understand how to make the best use of the time available. Inevitably service delivery and patient care will be positively impacted by successful time management, as processes and systems are implemented and maintained by a well organised team. The NHS Institute for Innovation and Improvement (2008) outlines three main career stages that have been identified and used throughout the MLCF. Stage 1 covers up to the end of undergraduate training, Stage 2 up to the end of postgraduate training and the final Stage 3 extends up to five years or equivalent post-specialist certification experience.

At undergraduate stage (Medical School), all medical students will be expected to attain the appropriate level of competence in management and leadership as defined by the Medical School curriculum (based on the General Medical Council's *Tomorrow's Doctors, 2004*).

During their Medical School training, students will have access to management and leadership learning opportunities within a variety of situations including peer interaction, clinical placement, and involvement with charities, social groups and organisations. All these situations can provide a medical student with the opportunity to develop management and leadership experience as they move from learner to practitioner upon graduation. A key part of personal effectiveness includes the practice of efficient time management principles.

At postgraduate stage the MLCF applies to doctors in training and practice i.e. during foundation years and for those in specialty training and non-specialist training posts.

The Institute emphasises that, as they consolidate their skills and knowledge in everyday practice, a doctor in training is very often the key medical person who relates to patients and other staff and experiences how day to day healthcare works in action. They are uniquely placed to develop experience in management and leadership through interaction with different people, departments and ways of working. This aids an understanding of a patient's healthcare experience and how the processes and systems of delivering care can be improved. Specific activities such as clinical audit and research also offer the opportunity to learn management and leadership skills. With all this comes the need to understand how a doctor's specialty and focus of care contributes to the wider healthcare system. With these broader responsibilities it is easy to understand how being able to identify priorities becomes paramount for doctors in training. At post-specialist certification stage the Framework applies to all senior doctors.

The end of the formal training period brings with it roles and responsibilities for delivering patient care, as well as in the wider healthcare system. This requires an understanding that all aspects of the team and hospital must function to standard for the system to work. Experienced doctors develop their abilities in management and leadership within their departments and practices, as well as working with colleagues in other settings and on research projects. As established members of staff, they are able to further develop their management and leadership abilities by actively contributing to the running of the organisation and the way care is provided generally. So, no matter what stage your medical career has reached, time management is a skill you need to extend.

The key principles of the MLCF are set out into the five main areas: personal qualities, working with others, managing services, improving services and setting direction. Successful time management impacts on all these areas. Each one is further broken down into four sub-sections.

The sub-groupings of Personal Qualities are:

- Acting with integrity
- Self development
- Self management
- Self awareness

It is easy to see from these headings how time management is appropriate to at least three of them. Improving your time management skills will be part of your continuing personal development and will play a key role in managing yourself. The first step to self improvement is self awareness and practising better time management will enable you to become aware of your bad habits or areas for development in this discipline.

The sub-groupings of Working with Others are:

- Working with teams
- Encouraging contribution
- Building and maintaining relationships
- Developing networks

As will be explored in later chapters these skills and abilities take time to develop and require practice. It will be necessary for you to make time to develop these skills, particularly as you progress in your career and become responsible for teams of people. The building and maintenance of relationships are important factors for doctors and a due amount of time must be allocated, whether it be spending time with juniors or acting as a positive influence with other team members.

The sub-groupings of Managing Services are:

- Managing performance
- Managing people
- Managing resources
- Planning

Managing people and their performance takes time, as does planning the correct resources for any service or project. Planning itself is time consuming and it is something often overlooked by busy doctors. When you already feel overwhelmed by a lack of time in which to achieve everything on your list, it may seem too challenging to have to find extra time in which to plan. However, you will find as you progress through this book, that planning will be a key part of organising your working week, and you will reap the benefits of allocating some time to this essential activity.

The sub-groupings of Improving Services are:

- Facilitating transformation
- Encouraging innovation
- Critically evaluating
- Ensuring patient safety

These principles focus heavily on the strategic aspect of a doctor's role and will affect you at some point in your medical career, even if that circumstance has not yet arisen. Strategic thinking requires a considerable amount of uninterrupted time, as does the creation of plans. Many operational responsibilities will have to be delegated in order for you to secure the time you need to focus on improving the services your department or team provides.

The sub-groupings of Setting Direction are:

- Evaluating impact
- Making decisions
- Applying knowledge and evidence
- Identifying the contexts for change

These are capabilities which require experience and practice, as setting direction is a fundamental leadership skill involving the competencies of strategic thinking and decision making. Poor decision making is one of the major causes of failure for time management, as it prevents progress on the commitments which require action. At first glance the MLCF appears to be relevant to management and leadership only, but as this chapter shows, it is a strong driver for the improvement of time management skills. In order for any doctor to achieve proficiency in these framework attributes it will be necessary to possess robust organisational skills.

As you become increasingly aware of the expectations placed upon you by this MLCF you will understand that, in addition to managing your time effectively, you will need to develop other management skills in parallel, such as the ability to set priorities for yourself and delegate work to others. You may need to develop your communication skills and an understanding of the importance of assertiveness, in the context of organising your time more effectively. This book will help you become aware of your current working practices, assist you in developing more productive disciplines and give you some tools which will help you identify your priorities and stick to them. The incorporation of these elements will also help you take a more proactive approach to crisis and prevent current stressful situations from re-occurring.

If you are feeling daunted by the expectations the Competency Framework places upon doctors, please understand that the number of skills you are expected to demonstrate is entirely dependent on where you are in your career. Medical students are, of course, expected to know and demonstrate fewer of the skills than doctors in training. Only senior doctors are expected to demonstrate the majority of the skills outlined. As doctors progress in their careers they will be exposed to greater opportunities where additional skills can be utilised. Managing your time successfully, however, is a skill which should be practised from the outset. A medical student would do well to organise his revision rota into a planned arrangement. Any doctor in training must make the most effective use of his or her time, given the almost overwhelming demands made by many different colleagues and patients. Senior doctors must be a role model for doctors in training, patients and all other healthcare practitioners as well as needing critical time for strategic responsibilities. As you can see there is a compelling case for anyone in medicine to manage time in a resourceful way.

Medicine is not alone in needing to face up to time management issues. Research has shown that wasted time in corporate organisations costs up to £80 billion each year which equates to 7% of Gross Domestic Product. The same research discovered that there was a general lack of leadership in these organisations and that their culture did not support effective time management. The purpose of this book is not to explore whether such a culture exists within medicine but to invite all doctors to proactively use the time they have in the most productive way, regardless of the prevailing environment.

To accommodate these immense pressures it is clear that profound changes are required. This book will offer you the chance to become more creative and view things from a different perspective. You already know the outcomes of your current working practices. Trying an alternative approach will lead to a different outcome. If it is not the one you want, then keep changing your approach until you achieve the success you seek.

Time management is not a difficult topic and yet it is still one of the most difficult skills to conquer for many doctors. Understanding why will be an extremely useful step forward. What is becoming evident is that tools and techniques are not enough. There must be an intangible factor and this is undoubtedly the commitment that is required from you to change the way you currently work. Only this adjustment will secure your success.

The emphasis on quality

In order for an organisation to perform at a consistently high standard, it depends upon the abilities of each employee. Your workplace is monitored continually for its efficiencies and the quality of patient care.

In recent years, for example, with the introduction in the UK of the NHS Plan and Lord Darzi's commitment to improve quality, there is an identified need for doctors to become much more personally effective within their environment. Doctors have great influence, more than they realise sometimes, but can be bewildered by the organisation they work within.

Now, more than ever, it is essential that you learn how to influence the system within which you work and use the time you have available to generate the greatest impact. Better time management skills will be a crucial factor for your personal effectiveness within medicine.

This workbook is going to give you the foundations of effective time management in the simplest way possible and the rest is up to you. Each chapter will begin with some aims and objectives and end with a personal development exercise, giving you the opportunity to put the theory into practice. All chapters end with a summary of the points covered.

Having read the above, you may decide that you only have a few tweaks to make, in which case feel free to skip chapters and try the exercises that you feel would really make a difference to you. For those of you, who feel helplessly sucked into a spiral of 'too much to do and not enough time, to do it,' read on.

References

European Working Time Directive (1998, 2003)
www.dh.gov.uk and www.healthcareworkforce.nhs.uk

The Academy of Medical Royal Colleges and the NHS Institute for Innovation and Improvement, *Medical Leadership Competency Framework* (2008)
www.institute.nhs.uk
(Can download the 80 page document in PDF format from this website)

General Medical Council, *Tomorrows Doctors* (1993, 2003)
http://www.gmc-uk.org/education/undergraduate/undergraduate_policy/tomorrows_doctors.asp

Workforce Review Team (1999)
http://www.wrt.nhs.uk/

Chapter 1   The need for personal effectiveness

Aims & objectives

In this chapter you will:

- Understand why personal effectiveness is necessary in modern medicine
- Discover the benefit of managing your time successfully
- Discover your time management profile
- Learn why being effective is critical for all doctors
- Understand how effective time management contributes to reduced stress levels
- Explore what can be managed
- Identify the impact of successful time management on your life
- Discover how committed you are to change

Why personal effectiveness is necessary in modern medicine

Within the context of *The Medical Leadership Competency Framework*, there is a clearly identified requirement for all doctors to become much more effective within medicine. There has been a definite shift away from exclusive focus on clinical excellence and an acknowledgement of additional skills which will help doctors achieve success in the overall delivery of services. Doctors need to communicate effectively with patients and peers. They need team working skills, knowing when to offer support and when to make a contribution for the over-riding good of the service. They need to be able to set direction for themselves and potentially other people and create goals and outcomes as well as being able to distribute workload and responsibilities in a fair and balanced manner. Greater insight into the priorities of the department so that the bigger picture of the overall service can be considered is paramount. Modern medicine is a very different place to that experienced by previous generations of doctors. These additional expectations of competencies bring greater pressures on individuals and the need for self-organisation is evident. Above all, excellent patient care is the ultimate target which is why all doctors are being actively encouraged to widen their focus and broaden their skill-set.

As mentioned in the introduction of this book, time management is now recognised as a fundamental capability at all levels of a medical career, as its influence on getting things done and on other people is far reaching. Doctors possess the potential for great influence but until they can manage their working day effectively, that influence will be diminished to a large extent.

The benefits of managing your time successfully

In addition to the many positive effects on your working life, there are personal benefits attached to managing your time more successfully. As you begin to organise your day into a meaningful structure your productivity will rise. Working to a pre-planned framework will allow you to attend to many more tasks because you will be paying closer attention to how you spend the hours in your working day. Many doctors report a lack of awareness around how much time they have available. They admit to not making the best of their available time because the only fixed items in their diary are their clinics. Other than those scheduled events, the diary is vague and many doctors describe the remaining time as being open to whichever pressing need arises first. By planning and consciously committing to undertake certain activities your output will rise and along with it your sense of confidence in your own abilities. As you regain control of your day your stress levels will reduce significantly and you become caught up in a positive cycle of effectiveness, confidence and the motivation to perpetuate the sequence.

Discover your time management profile

The first step to improving your personal effectiveness is to develop self awareness. Indeed it is one of the competencies mentioned in the 'Personal Qualities' section of the *Competency Framework.* Irrespective of this, no doctor can be expected to improve performance without first understanding where the deficiencies lie. Read the following descriptions of two doctors whose approach to personal organisation is very different and see who you identify most closely with.

A Typical Day for Dr Azri Kumar

Dr Kumar is a dedicated doctor. He prides himself on his excellent relationships with patients and they are most important to him. He cares deeply about their on-going treatment and always spends as much time as he can with each one. He does not aspire to be overly organised but does not consider this a problem because his main concern is being an excellent clinician for his patients. His days are usually unstructured and Dr Kumar works with a laissez faire style, becoming uncomfortable when anyone tries to plan his diary movements.

His clinics often over-run and he explains to the exasperated nursing staff that it is more important for the patient to be happy than to see everyone within a set timeframe.

He is meticulous about reading patient records and will often stay late into the evening to do so, in order for him to know every detail about a patient. Dr Kumar believes himself to be a great role model for his juniors. He acknowledges that he doesn't spend much time with the team, but justifies this in his mind because that was his experience as a junior and he does not believe it did him any harm. He takes pride in the fact that he often works late, a quality he admired in other senior doctors when he was a trainee.

His desk is always covered in paper and it is quite evident to others that he has difficulty finding anything. Dr Kumar is rather pleased with the image of the eccentric but excellent doctor he has created. However, many of his juniors do not share his opinion. They just find the impact of his disorganisation frustrating and time-consuming.

When he does get around to dealing with paperwork, Dr Kumar has not established a system for processing it and continually moves it around his desk as he is unsure how to deal with it. On a good day, when Dr Kumar feels able to concentrate for an hour or two, he chooses one particular pile of paperwork and works his way through. Unfortunately he is frequently interrupted, as Dr Kumar operates an open door policy. He cannot resist his ringing telephone and checks his e-mails at the start of his day and whenever he returns to his office.

Dr Kumar is late for many meetings. Being a senior doctor means that he is often asked for his opinion. As soon as he leaves his office someone stops him and asks him a question or wants a decision from him. He is pleased that people seek his view and he does not want to ignore them in order to get to his next meeting. When he does arrive he is happy to talk at length about any aspect of patient care and often leads the discussion that way, even when it is not the original topic. He prides himself on his ability to work relentlessly for his patients and they reward him by holding him in high regard.

Increasingly, however, Dr Kumar feels exhausted. Recently he has been suffering from severe headaches. To keep himself going during the day, he resorts to as many strong black coffees as he can fit in. He usually needs one before he can tackle the paperwork on his desk. When he returns home, it is often late at night. He is too tired to eat and falls into bed, next to his wife. Occasionally, she tells him how unhappy she is with their quality of life. Dr Kumar has no answers. He wishes she were more supportive of his career.

A Typical Day for Dr Susan Holden

Dr Holden is a committed senior doctor. In addition to her clinical duties she has a number of non-clinical responsibilities which she has to schedule into her diary each week. The perception of her colleagues is that she is a well organised individual who remains calm under pressure.

Having already planned her week, Dr Holden reviews her diary each morning, reminding her what is planned for the day ahead. She allocates the first 30 minutes to reading new e-mails and responds if she can do so within the time given.

Dr Holden then gets on with whatever activity she has planned during her non-clinic time. She manages a team of people and holds brief but regular meetings with each person, ensuring that they all get to spend some time with her. However, these are scheduled throughout her week so that she can manage her workload more easily. She chairs a team meeting each week, designed as a method of communicating relevant information to all parties.

She has developed systems and routines for her working day, built around clinical commitments. This includes keeping her office door closed when she wants to make important phone calls or concentrate on getting a specific job done. Everyone in the team understands that when Dr Holden's door is closed they must not enter. If there is an urgent requirement they do know that they can interrupt but usually knock before entering as a courtesy to Dr Holden.

If she needs to concentrate and does not want to be interrupted by unexpected events Dr Holden re-directs her telephone calls to the message service and closes her e-mail account. She reviews her e-mails three times a day so is not worried by closing the account for a while if she has something specific to address.

Dr Holden has a reputation of coping with the pressures and stress of the environment and never seems to lose her temper. She is rarely late for meetings and her desk is orderly although not free from paper. She does appear to utilise a filing system and can easily locate papers when she needs them.

She has recently been asked to head a major research project and is now reviewing her existing commitments to see which duties and responsibilities will have to be delegated so that she can make time for the research commitment each week in her diary.

Dr Holden is widely respected for her level headed approach and she appears to have clear sense of her priorities.

Which doctor do you relate to? Perhaps you share aspects with both approaches, beginning with good intentions but losing control at some point during the day.

If you are reading this book it is likely that you relate to Dr Kumar more closely. Do you see yourself in his behaviour? Do you share his beliefs about what it means to be a great doctor? Do you focus on your patients to the exclusion of most other things? Are you actually a hindrance to the secretaries who are waiting for the dictated notes you take so long to produce? Do you frustrate your nursing team who are highly organised but are prevented from being effective in their day-to-day work because you spend too long talking with patients? Think about how you currently spend your day. Whilst your time management practices may not present a problem for you personally, consider the impact of your behaviour on others around you. Do you spend your day running from clinics, to meetings, to ward rounds, to more meetings? Are you creating an impression of effectiveness or incompetence? Be careful. A desire to be seen as committed can be interpreted very differently.

If you are more junior perhaps you are unable to identify an appropriate person to whom you could delegate some of your activities. You may think it appropriate to keep your day unstructured so that you are available to meet the requests of senior colleagues.

No matter what stage you are at in your medical career, you have choices. You can choose to view things differently. You can choose to alter your beliefs about how many hours you are expected to work. Look around you. Do you have role models? Do you have colleagues who have clear, or clearer, desks than you? Do you know individuals who are able to delegate confidently? They are the effective time managers. There are individuals who have as much work as you, and face as many pressures as you do, but still manage to fit it all in and have a life outside work. If anyone springs to mind, observe them a little more closely from now on. How do they manage it? What do they say to people? It is likely they manage other people's expectations and are able to ask other people for help if they need it. They probably have good social lives and ensure that as much as possible is done during their working day so that they can meet their outside commitments. It is probably equally true that at no time is the care of their patients compromised or at risk. If they can do it, so can you.

If you want to work in a similar way to Dr Holden, consider what needs to change in order for that to happen. What do you need to do differently?

Remember that self-awareness is the key to change. You need to understand your personal strengths and weaknesses and develop yourself if you are to become more effective in your environment. There is less room in modern medicine for an exclusively patient focused clinician. Of course patient care is your ultimate aim but you will have to be proficient in a number of skills to deliver that excellent service to your patients.

Being effective is critical for all doctors

Think about all the things you need to accomplish as a doctor. At some point in your career you will need to create business cases to purchase equipment or hire extra resources. You will often find yourself in situations that require you to negotiate with others to achieve your outcomes. You may need to persuade and convince other people that your plan is the best one. You will definitely need to develop a strategy for the future and to make it inspiring enough that others are motivated to follow. The more senior you become the more you will be expected to manage a team of people, directing their actions in the most productive way for your service. You will be actively involved in the mentoring of junior staff. You will devise training plans and be expected to communicate frequently with your team. Above all you will be expected to defend them from unwarranted criticism and to support and praise them when they are performing well. You will attend senior level meetings and be involved with agreeing major contracts and service level agreements. As you can see, the more senior you become, the more you are drawn away from clinical responsibilities. You do not have to exclude them altogether but it is important that you understand what is expected of you when you hold a senior role. A lot of self-preparation is required and the earlier in your career that you can start, the better it will be for you. You need to be effective in your healthcare organisation as you will have many things to get done. There is a compelling argument for being able to organise yourself and your working day so that you do not become overwhelmed with all that you need to achieve.

The impact on stress levels

The other forceful reason for regaining control of your time relates to stress. As you know, stress does not need to be harmful but the term has come to be associated with a more negative connotation. People use the term stress to describe the feeling they have when it all seems too much, when they are overloaded and do not feel that they are able to meet all the demands placed upon them.

In relation to performance, there is an optimum point where you have enough pressure to perform, but not so much that you get overloaded. Everyone's optimum point is different and learning where yours is can be important.

In general, stress is related to both external and internal factors. External factors include your job, your relationships with others, your home and all the challenges, difficulties and expectations you have to deal with on a daily basis. Internal factors determine your body's ability to respond to, and deal with, the external stress-inducing factors. Internal factors which influence your ability to handle stress include your nutritional status, overall health and fitness levels, emotional well-being, and the amount of sleep and rest you get.

Excess stress can manifest itself in a variety of symptoms and these vary enormously among different individuals. Common physical symptoms often reported by those experiencing excess stress include sleep disturbances, muscle tension, headache, gastrointestinal disturbances and fatigue. Emotional and behavioural symptoms that can accompany excess stress include anxiety, mood swings, changes in eating habits and a loss of enthusiasm or energy. Poor time management can lead to the disturbances described above. Are you experiencing any of the symptoms?

It is also known that people under stress may have a greater tendency to drink and smoke excessively and grab an unhealthy snack, to be eaten on the go, than less-stressed colleagues. These unhealthy behaviours can further increase the severity of symptoms related to stress, often leading to an unhelpful cycle of symptoms and unhealthy habits.

It must be emphasised that the experience of stress is highly individualised. What constitutes overwhelming stress for one person may not be perceived as stress by another. Likewise, the symptoms and signs of poorly managed stress will be different for each person. Nevertheless, stress is a risk for doctors, whose patient care could be compromised as a result. Effective time management will dramatically reduce your stress levels as you begin to get things done, as planned and on time. Regaining a sense of control in your life will help you feel that you can manage your workload. Setting aside enough time to eat is important to your well-being. Many junior doctors believe that they should not take a break but this mind-set will not make an effective clinician. Conversely, it could affect objective judgement and concentration and the risk of mistakes is greater than before.

What can be managed?

Have you got any control over time? Not really. To focus your efforts on changing the clock will be futile. Time passes no matter what you do or do not do. It happens in spite of you. It is more helpful for you to focus your energies into changing how you manage the events and activities that occur each day. In other words, what you do with the time given rather than time itself. How you choose to spend each minute of each hour is up to you and completely within your control. If you were granted an extra two hours each day would you get more done? Or just have more time to waste? It is an interesting question and your answer will probably give you greater insight into the cause of your current dilemma. Perhaps you are not as effective as you would like because you do not manage your workload in a focused manner.

Personal effectiveness stems from managing events, activities and other people in the most productive way. For ease of reference, this book will continue to use the term time management throughout, but it will be more useful for you to move away from a desire to control time and to consider how you could manage the events and tasks that occur within each day. Consider how you need to manage other people in order to achieve what you need to do.

The impact of successful time management

Remember that regaining control of your workload creates a very favourable impression of you as a competent doctor who will earn the respect of those around you. Your reputation will grow in tandem with your organisational skills and you will reach the attention of influential individuals which may be very useful for your career. You will also benefit personally, as you should be able to regain a work/life balance and include other hobbies and interests in your life, making you a more rounded individual.

How committed are you?

In relation to the statements you have just read think about what needs to change. Have you developed un-resourceful habits which could do with being replaced? Have you been enjoying a martyred existence, complaining to everyone how hard you work? Have you gained their sympathy? Or have they dismissed you as they have witnessed your unwillingness to change? Being a martyr rarely earns respect so instead of continuing with a victim frame of mind, actively work out what you can do differently to improve your effectiveness. Nothing is more persuasive to the medical community than evidence, so think about what impression you currently create and what you need to change in order to create a much better impression of yourself as the kind of doctor that is expected in medicine today.

Exercise

To gain an insight into your stress levels and your ability to organise how you spend your time effectively, read through the following statements and make a note of the ones you relate to.

Common time management statements

'There aren't enough hours in the day.'

'I don't enjoy the job like I used to. I'm always running around trying to catch up.'

'No-one understands what it's like for doctors.'

'I try to stick to my to-do lists but it never works out that way.'

'I can't trust anyone else to do the job as well as me'

'By the time I've told someone else how to do it, it will have been quicker to do it myself.'

'I have no balance between my personal life and my working life. I just can't seem to manage the two.'

'I think and talk about work most evenings when I get home.'

'I often put things off but there is so much to do I am sometimes overwhelmed by it all.'

'If only I could stop the work coming in for a few days and just deal with what's on my desk at the moment, I could get back in control again.

'Of course, I'm stressed. But so is everyone else!'

'They don't understand. There really is too much to do.'

'We need more resources.'

Underline the statements you identify with. Taking each one in turn, consider what you can do to change the situation. Do you need to be more assertive and defend your right to take a break or leave at a reasonable hour? Do you need to be more organised? Are you easily distracted by outside interruptions and do you frequently put off those tasks which daunt you? There could be many reasons preventing you from making the most of the time you have. You need to discover them and work out how things could change for the better. How are you going to become more effective? Write down an action statement for each one beginning with 'I'. It is important you take ownership of the things you wish to change.

Summary

- The skill of managing time is critical for all doctors.

- Modern medicine requires doctors to accomplish much more than spending time with patients.

- Self-awareness is the first step to become personally effective in medicine.

- Are you a Dr Kumar or a Dr Holden?

- As influential individuals, all doctors are expected to negotiate, persuade, assert, organise and manage people and resources.

- Successful time management reduces stress levels.

- It is possible to regain control of one's day so that workloads become manageable.

- Effective time managers gain a deserved reputation of competence and calmness; they are individuals who react well to pressure.

- Everything is a choice and you can choose to manage your activities in a more organised way.

Chapter 2 Who or what steals your time?

Aims & objectives

In this chapter you will find out:

- How your unconscious habits plague your day-to-day effectiveness

- Which areas could do with more focus?

- The problems of 'To Do' lists

- The enemy of getting things done – procrastination

- Who sabotages your time and efforts?

- The main factors of your time management problems

- How technology has made a significant impact on medical workloads

It is likely you feel that if it were not for your overwhelming workload you would be able to manage your time with ease. Most of the individuals who struggle to organise their activities effectively will often state that no-one understands what it is like for them and that there is too much work to do and too few people. That is probably true to some extent, which makes the need for some time management techniques that work all the more necessary. However, more often than not a lack of time is not really the issue. It is the inability to use the time you have effectively that is the underlying issue. If your workload seems insurmountable the more personally organised you can become, the better. At least trying to apply some sort of order to your day will yield greater results than not trying at all. The good news is to realise that you are not alone in your struggles. This chapter attempts to identify some of the more generic issues facing many doctors in modern medicine.

Daily habits – the thieves of time

When individuals start to take a closer look at their working practices, some interesting strategies come to light. Many people have routine ways of starting their day at work. They have been doing the same thing for so long that the activities have become habits and are no longer noticed. Whilst habits can be extremely useful as they require little mental effort, some can work against you. For example, a very common unconscious habit for many is the obligatory morning cup of coffee or tea. Having arrived at your hospital or health centre how long is it before you are heading for the coffee machine or kitchen? You probably feel that without your first coffee you will not be fully awake. You may feel that you need it just to get going. As you read this you may wonder what could be the harm in making a drink? After all it doesn't take long. In reality, what may seem like a two minute activity can often turn into a ten minute conversation with a colleague who happens to be carrying out the same routine habit to start their day. You may not even make it to the coffee point before being stopped by someone who needs to ask you a question or wants 'a moment' of your time. A moment? How long is a moment? If you manage to get to the machine without being stopped, it is likely someone will stop you on your return. This may not happen every morning and the amount of time you lose will vary depending upon the other person and the complexity of their request or issue and that isn't really the concern. What is crucial is that you will probably lose the first thirty minutes of your day before you even begin to turn your thoughts to your own workload.

When you finally do make it back to your desk you will probably automatically deploy unconscious habit number two. Like Dr Kumar you will decide to log onto your e-mail account and check for new mail. E-mail was a revolutionary communication tool when it was introduced. Over the last fifty years the traditional method of communicating, that of face to face, has changed in favour of telephone or e-mail interactions. When e-mail systems were first adopted as a business tool they were heralded as a way of improving the speed of communication. The reality may have evolved somewhat differently to the concept. The impact of e-mail, as a method of communicating, on time management has been enormous. It is estimated that individuals now spend one to two hours of each working day reading and writing e-mail. A real problem for many is that they receive e-mail that has no relevance to them and this is often via the 'copy to' option. Some communicators only feel comfortable when they have shared the information with as many people as possible. As a means of doing so, no-one would disagree that e-mail is not the most efficient way. However, this habit of distributing so much, to so many can be infuriating and time-wasting. How many e-mails do you receive which are of little significance or interest to you? E-mail can only be an effective means of communication provided it is used sensibly. A real hindrance of e-mail for you is that you will have to read most of them in order to find out whether their content is of any value to you. Whether you view e-mail as a positive or negative element of your time management system, it is part of modern life and here to stay. The challenge for all doctors will be to ensure that it is they who manage their e-mails and not the other way around.

A third unconscious habit which may be used by some people is to put off the start of the working day by having a chat with colleagues. This will be particularly true of a Monday morning when there is much to talk about after the weekend. This book is not suggesting that you stop conversing with your colleagues altogether. However, consider the impact that these conversations are having on you. Are they stopping you from getting on with your work? Could there be a better time to talk, such as during a lunch break? Could they be shortened, however enjoyable they are? Socialising with the team is important, but not if it is at the expense of work that is being neglected and that could cause you more stress in the long run. Think of your options and remember your commitment to change.

Lack of focus

Successful time management requires a commitment to change and the focus and motivation to maintain that change. For many people a lack of focus lies at the heart of their time management struggles. In the earlier example, the problem for Dr Kumar was his narrow focus. He needed to see the bigger picture, rather than concentrating solely on patient care. It is an admirable intention but is not useful within modern medicine which requires doctors to be more than good clinicians. Doctors need to be excellent communicators, highly organised to cope with heavy workloads, be aware of changing priorities and to cope with frequent changes to policies and targets. Flexibility is a useful skill to acquire especially as doctors are also required to develop management skills, in order to deploy valuable resources within strict budgets. With so many responsibilities the need for focus is clear. All doctors must concentrate on the essentials of the role and the requirements of their environment. Without this too many doctors fall prey to dealing with issues as they arise without any clear idea of what they should be focusing on. Take a moment to consider the areas where you could apply more focus in your working life. What is stopping you from being that way now?

The drawbacks of To Do lists

Some doctors and healthcare professionals make lists of things to do and consider that to be effective time management. The problem with a list is that it rarely diminishes. It just gets longer and longer as more items are added after another interrupted day. It provides no guarantee that anything on the list will be done. Lists can actually increase stress levels as they visibly become longer.

They can even become one of your negative habits, as the very act of writing them each day, successfully stops you from beginning your important tasks and insidiously steals the time available to you. The biggest problem of all with a 'To Do' list is that it has no sense of priority. Usually people create their lists from a brainstorm. Any outstanding action is written down, as it emerges from the brain and the 'To Do' list becomes a record of unrelated activities with no indication of what should be tackled first. It is difficult to develop a sense of focus and purpose when there is little indication of what to concentrate on. 'To Do' lists will undoubtedly help you feel busy and efficient, simply because you have been able to capture all the unactioned tasks but it is unlikely that they will help you become effective.

It is fair to say that 'To Do' lists make a useful starting point. In earlier generations of time management theories they were heralded as the foundation of personal organisation. For most people it is less stressful to write actions down then it is to carry them around in their heads. However, the problem remains that a list of activities is not enough to solve time management issues. How do you know which task to do first? How will you know what to focus on? A later chapter will show you how to take the list one step further so that it becomes a useful aid to managing your workload.

A formidable enemy of good time management – procrastination

The title of this chapter asks who or what steals your time. This would imply that external factors are solely to blame. It would be naive to ignore your own role in this situation, you may be the main reason why you are not getting things done on time. Procrastination is a critical enemy of effective time management. It means to put off a task or action until a later time. The word comes from the Latin word *procrastinatus*: *pro-* (forward) and *crastinus* (of tomorrow). Procrastination can be described as a coping mechanism for dealing with the anxiety associated of starting a particular task or project. Although it is normal for people to delay difficult or dreaded tasks to some degree it doesn't actually help. Many people feel stressed at the thought of doing a particular task or activity. For example, imagine you have been asked by a senior colleague to make a presentation at an important meeting in a month's time. You are expected to prepare a 60 minute talk with slides and to speak confidently about a topic of which you have limited knowledge. It is likely that the prospect of giving this presentation is daunting for you and the necessary preparation will require a lot of effort on your part. You now have a choice about how you wish to handle this assignment. You may perceive it as a great career opportunity and a chance to create a good impression of yourself to your senior colleagues. With that in mind you will probably embark upon the task with energy and excitement. Or you may feel very anxious about the event and decide to put off any work associated with it for as long as possible. You may even believe that in doing so you can relieve your anxieties and put the event out of your mind for at least another 3 weeks. What you will discover, however, is what effective time managers already know. When you procrastinate you actually increase your feelings of stress, not diminish them. The feeling of fear never leaves you and becomes an added burden for you to carry around during the forthcoming month.

All the time you are putting off the preparation of that future task or project you will also experience feelings of guilt. You know you should be getting on with it but you cannot face it. This is another common reaction to putting things off and, as is the case with stress, feelings of guilt do not go away until the task is complete.

Time management tip

The only way to relieve feelings of guilt and anxiety about not doing an action is to start the very thing you do not want to do.

Please remember that whenever you procrastinate you are not being as productive as you should. This loss of personal productivity will impact on all areas of your medical role and responsibilities. You will be less effective as a result and this approach cannot be sustained as a long term strategy. You will create a crisis for yourself and for those around you who rely on your timely execution of duties. As the well known saying goes, 'do not put off until tomorrow what you can do today'. Make a commitment to start and summon your determination. It does not matter how small the first action is, as long as you do it. It will help you break through the barrier of resistance.

How do you feel about starting a project that will take many months to complete? Some doctors are daunted by very complex undertakings or those activities which will take a long time. It can be difficult to decide where to begin and to estimate how long something will take. This lack of clarity can be enough for individuals to put off starting something indefinitely but can only lead to a crisis situation when there is too much to do in the little time left. Later chapters will show you how to overcome your resistance and get started.

Junior doctors run a real risk of incurring the disapproval of seniors who will be unimpressed at their inability to get on with things. Senior doctors who procrastinate will develop a reputation of creating chaos amongst the team and will not be viewed as effective leaders.

In summary, procrastination may result in a number of negative impacts such as personal stress, feeling guilty, a loss of personal effectiveness and the disapproval of others for not fulfilling one's responsibilities or commitments. These feelings will not reduce until some action is taken. If the task continues to be deferred until a later date, these feelings will compound and promote further procrastination. Chronic procrastination could lead to serious problems for doctors and could cast doubt on their capabilities.

Sometimes the opposite is true and procrastination arises because of too little pressure. Anxiety can create motivation to get on with a task and if there is a distant deadline it may create a perception that no action is required until later. It is the sense of urgency that is often the catalyst for action. Therefore, tasks or projects will often be put off until the deadline looms into view. As you can imagine this is a high risk strategy which will yield inconsistent results. Sometimes the task will be completed successfully. More often than not another unanticipated event will also arise, forcing the individual to undertake both commitments and give neither the full attention required. This way of working is draining and unsustainable, not to mention stressful. If you want to become an effective and organised manager of your daily activities you will get on with a task, or part of it, if you have time enough available to do so. You will not be lulled into a false sense of not needing to attend to a task, because it has a remote deadline. You will understand that getting on with something while you have time available will help you manage any unexpected delays or problems nearer the deadline.

There are several ways in which you steal your own time each day, such as not being aware of your negative habits, not having focus and continually making 'to do' lists. These are all forms of procrastination, as they successfully prevent you from getting on with your daily tasks.

Who else is a saboteur of your time?

However, for many doctors, other people are also a significant factor. It is worth considering now who are the saboteurs of your working day? Is it your patients? Do some require more of your time than you can realistically give? Or do you work with more dominant personalities and find them occupying your time which could be put to better use elsewhere? Perhaps you are the only saboteur, allowing yourself to be distracted by many of the reasons cited already in this chapter.

For most people, it is a mixture of all three factors. Your unconscious and destructive habits, as well as an inability to deal with other people who continually make demands on your time, make for a very weak approach to managing time and events that occur within it.

Two main factors of time management problems

Being unable to say 'no' is the biggest obstacle to becoming organised. It will not matter how many lists you have made or how many priorities you have identified. If you cannot say 'no' to unexpected requests, then you will never keep control of how you spend your time. There are many reasons that doctors give for not being able to do this.

As the requirement for assertive communication is so essential for personal effectiveness in medicine and such a challenge for many doctors, an entire chapter will be devoted to this skill later in the book. For now, work out whether this is a problem for you and contributes to your difficulties with managing your commitments. It will be a poor doctor who, at appraisal time, tells his senior colleague proudly that he or she has successfully helped colleagues achieve their annual objectives but not had time to attend to the achievement of his or her own.

Another problem for doctors within the realm of other people is the inability to delegate. Feelings of guilt often arise when asking other people to help out. Yet surely this is part of teamwork? In order to delegate successfully the perception needs to shift to a more productive view. Instead of feeling guilty about burdening another person, it would be far more productive to realise that trainees need to develop their knowledge and skills and cannot do that unless they are given specific tasks. They need you to delegate or they will not progress properly in their training. Doctors who are not yet team leaders can still delegate to their peers in the team. This is not being lazy, unless it is specifically done for that reason. It is being mature enough to put the needs of the patients first and to understand that the service provided is more important than worrying about ensuring that each team member has exactly the same amount of work. All healthcare practitioners are busy and that will not change. Putting patient care first may create an appropriate environment for delegation.

As delegation is a key management and personal effectiveness skill and critical to time management a later chapter will explore the resistance many doctors feel about delegating. It will also provide guidance on the best ways of delegating which may help you overcome your natural reluctance.

Guilt is a real feeling experienced by many doctors, when they want to say no to other people or when they need to delegate and this feeling can be experienced by any doctor, no matter where they are in their career. The advice of this book is to learn to deal with those feelings and overcome them as soon as possible. To be effective you cannot be a slave to your emotions. You have to be confident in your reasons for saying no or for delegating. Handle your discomfort and then get on with the job you need to do. To advise you to 'get over it' may sound flippant but it is actually good advice. To be successful you have to overcome your self-imposed barriers or you will never fulfil your potential to be an excellent doctor, with many skills, both clinical and non-clinical.

Interruptions and unexpected events are frequently cited by doctors as huge time wasters. These happen to everyone in their working lives and the interesting element to note is that unexpected events are anticipated every day. Therefore, they are expected. Not knowing when the interruptions or unexpected events will occur seems to make them unmanageable for many doctors. The trick, of course, is to expect the unexpected and create time in the day to allow for some sort of interruption. Becoming effective at time management means anticipating these incidents and working out a plan of action, should the unexpected actually happen. It is possible to manage anything when it is anticipated and planned for. Only a haphazard response will undermine you.

The advance of technology has also had a huge impact on how we manage our workload and can have a detrimental effect on some individuals. We live in a world of 24-hour communications and it is easy to be drawn into viewing your e-mails as they arrive or answering the telephone whenever it rings. The onset of Blackberry handsets only makes it easier to take your work home with you. Some hospital services feel that the introduction of Blackberry's would be an ideal way of using the technology available to enhance team communication. Elusive senior doctors could be found more easily and nurses already on a ward could be asked to remain there to deal with another patient. As long as these suggested strategies are thought through and the full impact on working lives is explored, then technology can be utilised successfully. Often though, a solution to a breakdown in

communications can lead to a problem in the time management field, as
the individuals concerned start to feel threatened by their perceived feeling
of constantly being available.

Exercise

A valuable way of becoming more aware of how you spend your time
is to complete a time log. Keep a record of your actions as they happen.
Record how long you spend with each patient, how long each telephone
call takes and how long your breaks are. Record everything you do and
keep a log for three days. No day will be the same but by capturing your
activities over a longer period you should be able to recognise a pattern
of working practice.

You can create your own time log on the PC or simply keep a list of your
actions with times and duration noted against each one.

Use this sample as a guide:

Time	Activity	Duration
8.30	Coffee	5 minutes
8.35	Logged on to e-mail	5 minutes
8.40	Read new e-mails	20 minutes
9.00	Answered telephone call	13 minutes
9.15	Spoke with colleague	10 minutes
9.25	Preparing for ward round	20 minutes

Try not to leave the completion of your time log until the end of your
day. You will not remember accurately and will estimate the time taken
to do things and you will probably under estimate the duration of most
activities. Recording activities as they happen is the only way to gain
true insight into your habits and behaviour and will identify who or what
steals your time.

Summary

• Unconscious habits, such as the early morning coffee and chatting to colleagues plague your day-to-day effectiveness. Seemingly short activities add up during the day.

• A lack of focus hinders effective time management. Until you know what to concentrate on your attempts at being organised will remain haphazard.

• 'To Do' lists are helpful but are not the whole answer. They are often a collection of randomised thoughts and can grow in size rather than reduce.

• You may be your worst enemy regarding the effective use of your time. Resisting complex or unpleasant tasks increases stress levels. Do not put things off.

• Other people may sabotage your time and efforts.

• Saying no and an inability to delegate may be the main factors in your time management problems.

• The expansion of technology has made a significant impact on medical workloads. Managed properly, they can be useful tools of communication. However, you must work out how to use them to your advantage if you are to utilise them properly.

Chapter 3   Take a closer look

Aims & objectives

In this chapter you will:

- Find out who has to change – you or your colleagues?

- Take at a look at your working practices through the eyes of your senior. Define your real role, not the one you are doing now

- Understand the importance of time management during clinics

- Apply the 80/20 rule and your personal prime time and decide which activities you should be doing during it

- Use transition time wisely

- Decide which activities must stop now

- Learn how to break rapport

- Design your ideal working day

If you have read the introductory chapters of this book you will now have a better understanding of why it is essential that doctors become more effective in managing their time. If you have read chapter two you may have started a process of reflection and are becoming aware of the possible reasons why you have not been managing your time efficiently.

You may have identified closely with some of the statements made in chapter one and be forming some idea of actions that may help you change. Chapter two may have given you closer insights into what stops you from gaining control of your day, and being able to leave work on time with all your tasks complete. If you have kept a record of your activities, using a time log for two or three days, you probably have a very good idea of how you manage your time! All of this is useful information. Until you are aware of how you behave and how you are contributing to your problems with managing time, you cannot hope to resolve them.

Chapter three continues this process and invites you to take a closer look at your unique approach to your work. Whilst you may have been able to relate to some of the general issues suggested in the previous chapter, every person is different and will have problems of their own. This provides a real opportunity to assess your individual situation and thought processes. At the same time this chapter will offer some immediate suggestions for improvement to give you some encouragement. The remaining chapters will provide you with tools and techniques for alleviating your immediate problems and for establishing organised systems to maintain your effectiveness in the long term. You will learn how to make the best use of the time available and reduce your stress levels so that you can be the best doctor for your patients and a valued colleague.

Who needs to change?

What do you need to be more honest about? What has to change in order for you to become a more effective doctor? If your problems really do lie with other people, you will need to work out how you are going to manage them in the future. You need to devise a plan of action that will help you anticipate the requests of others and how you wish to respond. For very assertive individuals you may decide that a strategy of negotiation is required. Or you may need to practice saying no to colleagues and feel comfortable with that.

Maybe you have a desire to be seen as helpful and reliable. This encourages you to take on more work than you can handle. It may take precedence over your own work. If this is the issue the problem lies with you rather than other people and needs to be rectified immediately. It is a destructive habit and one that will overwhelm you. This book does not advocate never helping other people but it advocates that you choose when to be helpful and when you genuinely have the time.

If you are in the habit of taking on work that stimulates or interests you, control your tendencies to volunteer for this kind of work until you have addressed your priorities.

It is important that you work out your weak areas in terms of your responsibilities. When using your time logs pay attention to your working habits and identify those elements of work that you allow yourself to neglect, perhaps because they are less appealing to you. Be honest about these and understand that you have to do them. You may have to force yourself but once they are done you can then focus on the tasks you prefer.

All of this is within your control, but you have to make a commitment to do things differently.

Become your senior

One way that may help to give you greater insight into your time management flaws is to become your senior colleague for a moment. Scrutinise yourself through the eyes of the person you report to. What do you see? Does your leader consider you to be a reliable member of the team? Or do you give an alternative impression? Could it be possible that your senior colleague sees you as a rather ineffectual individual who appears to be overwhelmed by the workload? You may appear out of your depth just because you currently have not developed the ability to focus on the task in hand and get on with it. For whatever reason, you continue to switch from one task to another, never actually completing anything. It doesn't take long to create the impression of chaotic working practices.

Your real role versus your current role

All job roles have something called discretionary time and response time built into them. Response time refers to the activities over which you have little control. Your clinics and ward rounds would be examples of response time. Time management techniques have less impact on this time because you do not control it. These events are scheduled and you have to attend. However, it is true to say that some doctors prefer to spend the majority of their time engaged in these activities, spending far longer on them than is necessary. Discretionary time is the term given to that part of each day which is within your control. During these times you have the flexibility to decide what you are going to do. You probably have no formal commitments in the diary and can choose how you spend the time. This is where enormous amounts of valuable time can be wasted because there is no focused activity and no advance planning. There is often a perception that senior doctors have far more discretionary time than junior doctors. Whatever the reality, everyone has some element of discretionary time available to them which could be used much more effectively.

Consider your current role. Work out how much time is responsive and how much is discretionary. Do not work this out based on your current practices. Work it out as if you were a human resources manager and define it on the basis of what it should be, i.e. if the role was being executed as it was originally intended. For example, perhaps a common amount of discretionary time for doctors is forty per cent and response time is sixty per cent. For you it may be different but be brutally honest. If you are honest with yourself you probably know that, in reality, there is more discretionary time but, because of the way you work, that discretionary time has reduced significantly. Whatever the case please view the discretionary time as an opportunity for improvement. This is where the time management techniques in this book will be most effective. However, if you maintain your focus in team meetings and ward rounds, you will also notice a substantial improvement in the response time areas of your job.

Clinical time management

It can be very difficult to manage your time during clinics and ward rounds. This may be due to an inability to manage talkative patients, or perhaps your colleagues also suffer from poor time management and cannot complete tasks in an appropriate length of time. You can have a great deal of influence with your patients. Many doctors who report time management issues with patients go on to describe how they invite patients to contact them at any time with queries or concerns. These same doctors operate an open door policy to patients and invite them to drop by whenever they need to. You can immediately identify the problems this will create. Just as you are about to start writing a complex report that requires time and applied effort, a patient appears or the telephone rings. Your report gets put to one side again. It is perfectly acceptable to change that policy and be clear to others about when you can be available and when you cannot.

It may be harder for you to influence senior colleagues who are poor time managers but if you are able to explain the impact on you and other members of the team when these events over-run, you may be able to influence your seniors more than you realise. Some doctors enjoy spending the majority of their time with patients but do not enjoy recording their notes. This activity is often deferred until the next day. However, the impact of doing so has far reaching consequences. Secretaries and other support staff have to wait for the notes to be dictated and given to them to transcribe. Is it fair to force someone else to stay late because you could not organise yourself? Administrative staff are often highly organised and will become extremely frustrated at not being able to maintain their schedule of work because of a shortcoming on your part.

Your colleagues who need the information as part of the handover may also be impacted by your lack of attention to detail. A high standard of patient care can be compromised if the information is not available in a timely manner. Think of the team as a whole. Could your improved time management have a positive impact on them? It is highly likely that it will. Returning to your discretionary time, what has happened to this? Have you allowed it to reduce because of your inability to manage your day? If you keep saying yes to extra responsibilities, or allowing yourself to be interrupted by other people, you will never get on top of your workload. You must be stricter and claw back your discretionary time.

Write down, day by day, all of the fixed commitments you have such as your ward rounds, any regular meetings, essentially all the things you cannot get out of. Now review how much time is left in each day. This simple exercise is often a very powerful one. When you can see your day written down on paper you will frequently see that it is less crammed than it currently feels. Many doctors have expressed surprise and relief at seeing, for the first time, just how many hours are not committed to fixed activities. How you choose to spend the remaining hours will be up to you but the first step is to realise you have more discretionary time than you think.

Identify a role model if you can. Who do you know who seems just as busy as you, but rarely shows signs of stress, seems to leave on time most days and is able to get through their workload without too much trouble. It will help you to observe them a little more closely. What is their approach to their work? How do they handle other people? If they are colleagues ask them! Perhaps they can help you improve your own time management strategies.

Some doctors prefer to focus on one task and do not allow themselves to be distracted by anything else until that task is complete. Others prefer to break down various tasks and projects into step by step processes and complete a series of steps for each one. You will find your own preferred way of working. The important thing is, having identified it, that you persevere with it. Remember you will need determination in order to create a more productive habit. It usually takes a month to foster a new habit and during that time you will have to apply yourself with a great deal of concentration but after that you will find your new ways of working become easier and more natural.

Not knowing how the time is spent is the main problem for doctors. Without that essential knowledge it is impossible to rectify. Planning becomes impossible and activities cannot be measured. It is hoped that the introduction of a time log will provide that much needed clarity and offer the opportunity to create plans of action and measure your success.

The 80/20 rule

In 1906, Italian economist Vilfredo Pareto created a mathematical formula to describe the unequal distribution of wealth in his country when he noted that twenty percent of the people owned eighty percent of the wealth. About forty years later, Quality Management pioneer, Dr. Joseph M. Juran recognised a similar principle which he called the "vital few and trivial many" which meant that twenty per cent of something is always responsible for 80 percent of the results. This became known as Pareto's Principle.

In Juran's initial work he identified twenty percent of the defects causing eighty percent of the problems but the principle can be applied in many contexts. Project Managers, for example, know that twenty percent of the work (the first 10 percent and the last ten percent) consume eighty percent of time and resources.

Successful time managers understand that focusing on twenty percent of activities will yield eighty percent of results. The value of the Pareto Principle for doctors is that it serves as a daily reminder to focus on the twenty per cent of tasks that matter and that enable the biggest results. The challenge for doctors is to identify and focus on those things. If something in the schedule has to slip, make sure it does not form part of that twenty percent of high yield activities.

As part of this process of taking a closer look at your day to day practices, work out how you can apply Pareto's Principle. Review everything you do each day and decide which activities bring you the greatest results. Make a commitment to focus on those each day.

In addition to identifying your most productive activities, return to your time log and identify your personal prime time. Consider at which points of the day you feel you are at your best for handling different types of work. For example, for work that requires research, do you feel more able first thing in the morning or would mid-afternoon suit you better? When do you feel you could most effectively handle the routine work? Work out how much you can get done when you are working well. Divide your day into morning, afternoon and evening and play to your strengths.

Now combine the two by reviewing your 20 per cent activities and deciding when you could most productively deal with them. Not every day will work out perfectly as some of your response time may clash with your prime time. However, do what you can and move commitments in your diary if that is possible. Find out and ask. Become a proactive time manager and do not give in to negative assumptions that things cannot change. You will never know until you try. Part of taking back control of your working and personal life is to take control of how you spend your time. Start talking to other people about how you could work more effectively. They may be impressed enough to accommodate your request.

Using transition time

This is time spent commuting to and from work or in situations when you are forced to wait for someone or something else. This is often perceived as dead time and of little value. However, effective time managers regard transition time as an invaluable resource because they understand that these vacant time slots can be utilised in many productive ways. For example, e-mails can be answered if you have the technology to do so. There are many portable devices available to assist with this. You can also use transition time to catch up with essential reading, either for research or to keep yourself up-to-date in your field. Another valuable use of transition time is to plan ahead and even more critically it provides the space to think, something that doctors believe they have little time for and do not do enough. All effective time managers allow themselves time to think, so that they can plan and avoid a reactionary, crisis approach to their work.

Work out now how much transition time you have each day and how you could use it to your advantage.

Which activities must stop?

Take a closer look at your current activities. What are you doing that needs to stop? When you scrutinise yourself properly you may be realising that you spend far too much of your day talking, whether that be to patients or colleagues. You may realise that you allow others to talk to you too much and spend more time than you should listening to the problems or woes of others. You may be the one that everyone confides in, the one who provides a shoulder to cry on. Despite the fact that this may make you feel valued, this approach can prove to be a burden. You cannot get through your tasks and duties while other people continue to take advantage of your good nature and sit at your desk off-loading their worries. Try and find a balance. Explain to your colleagues or patients that you have to meet a deadline and offer them an alternative time to talk. For colleagues it may be more appropriate to speak with them during a lunch break. Patients will require an empathetic but firm strategy. People around you must learn that you are not always available to them and after a few conversations about arranging a suitable time they will get the message and their unexpected appearances will diminish. You will probably feel uncomfortable at the change initially but keep reminding yourself of all the tasks you can progress as a result. Being a good listener will not help you achieve your annual objectives so do not give into the temptation of ego and return to your old ways in your desire to be wanted or liked.

The benefits of breaking rapport

The previous chapter explored the possibility that other people make it difficult for you to manage your time and could be a reason why you are unable to get on with your work. For some doctors having assertive conversations are uncomfortable. They feel guilty at turning patients away who need to talk and find themselves unable to break away despite knowing there are other tasks which require attention. If you can relate to this you will be relieved to note that conversations can be cut short in ways that do not offend. The most successful method is called breaking rapport. Rapport is one of the most important characteristics of unconscious human interaction. It is commonly described as being "in sync" with, or being "on the same wavelength" as the person with whom you are talking. Being able to build rapport is a critical skill for doctors as it is at the heart of all successful communication. It is possible to build rapport by maintaining eye contact with the other person and also by sharing common experiences or demonstrating an attentive interest in what the other person has to say.

Sometimes, however, it is entirely appropriate to break rapport and create a disconnection in the relationship between the two parties. Looking away is one of the most powerful ways to do so and starts to signal to the other party that it is time to stop talking. With colleagues you can also begin to pack away your papers or glance at your watch to indicate that you have another appointment. Other people read these signs very quickly and will often apologise for keeping you. You can smile and offer an apology, if it makes you feel better, whilst rising from your desk and gesturing your guest to the door. They will follow you without question and will not take offence. At no point do you need to become aggressive or be rude. You need to be firm and take control of the situation because you remember how much you have to do today. Being assertive is about defending your rights and in these situations you have every right to get on with your work.

The ideal day

This chapter has invited you to scrutinise your unique approach to your working day and to identify areas of improvement. As a way of drawing to a close, it would be useful to gain some motivation for change. Take a moment and reflect on your ideal working day. Try and imagine yourself working at your best. You will probably see yourself smiling and relaxed, dealing with your patients in an efficient but attentive manner and moving onto the other tasks which require your attention. You may feel motivated, in control and enjoying the fact that you know what has to be done and you have planned accordingly.

This may sound a little strange as a time management technique but what you are doing is training your mind. You are re-programming yourself for success. When you can see and hear the future and connect to positive feelings associated with it, you are effectively training yourself to become that person. It is a useful way of determining what you are aiming for. When you experience those feelings for real you will know that your transformation is happening and you will gain the confidence to continue. Picture yourself working on your priorities and having the strength of mind to defer unimportant activities or delegate them to other people if that is appropriate.

Adopt an objective perspective and become a time & motion consultant. This business efficiency technique is designed to reduce the number of motions in performing a task in order to increase productivity and reduce fatigue. While it may not be possible to do this for every task, look for efficiencies within your own working practices and those of the team as a whole. Be as detached as possible. Could improvements be made? Could traditional ways of working be changed so that time and money are saved or patient care improved? Look closely: what you discover may surprise you.

If things are to change for the better you must adopt smarter ways of working. If you had 26 hours in each day instead of 24 would you get any more done? Not if you continue to work as you do now. You would squander the extra time because without focus, motivation and determination, you will not have the energy you need to get on with what needs to be done. You would simply take longer to do your tasks or you would feel relaxed at having more time and put the task or project off for even longer. What you need is a system for progress, a system that drives you on, regardless of the people or events surrounding you.

What systems do you have in place currently? You will need a system for determining priorities. You will need a system for handling the paperwork that reaches your desk, preferably one that enables you to handle paper only once. You will require a personal system that enables you to remain focused and assertive with others when they try to distract you or persuade you to take on extra work. In the forthcoming chapters you will discover more and more compelling reasons for taking back control of the events in your life and work out a plan to get everything done on time. You will find the necessary motivation to hold assertive conversations with colleagues and patients because you will fully understand your priorities. It is only when you are fully informed that you can make meaningful decisions about how you wish to conduct your day.

Exercise

Work out how much discretionary and responsive time you should have in your role. Now work out what the reality is for you today. If you have far less discretionary time than you know the role should have, think about what you need to do in order to re-dress the balance. Write down a list of possible actions. When you have done this, consider the action or option which appeals the most. It may appeal because it is the easiest action or because you know it will have the greatest impact on your time management. The choice is yours but be honest with yourself and be strict. Implement an action that will start to give you back the discretionary time that the role contains but that you have lost. Do not be despondent. Take small steps, one at a time. Any change is better than no change.

Another self awareness exercise for you to try is to work out your prime time. As suggested in this chapter, pay attention to your energy levels and match the different kinds of tasks you need to complete to your prime time. Practice this for a few days and see if you are able to reduce your workload. If you are a morning person, tackle a more challenging task here. If you successfully complete it you will feel energised for the rest of the day. If you know that you are not at your best during the late afternoon, avoid the tasks that make mental demands of you. Work smarter and play to your strengths.

Summary

- Becoming aware of how you spend your time and your behaviour with other people is the only way to make necessary improvements.

- Looking at yourself through the eyes of your senior will afford you useful insights. What impression are you creating about yourself to others?

- Decide how much discretionary and response times your role contains. You have the greatest influence over your discretionary time.

- Time management techniques are less influential during clinic time but not ineffectual. You may be spending longer than you should with each patient.

- Work out your prime times. When are you most productive and what tasks should you be focusing on during those times?

- Use any transition time wisely.

- Look at your activities through the eyes of your senior. Apply the 80/20 rule and drop the activities which yield the least results.

- Breaking rapport is a useful way of discouraging unwanted visitors.

- Picture your ideal day at work.

- Look for efficiencies and be prepared to make drastic changes to working practices.

- Develop systems for success.

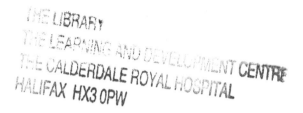

Chapter 4 Setting priorities

Aims & objectives

In this chapter you will:

- Learn about the importance of setting priorities
- Learn the various options for prioritising available
- Develop a clear sense of what has to be done
- Deal with the present situation to regain a sense of control
- Be able to separate actions into important and immediate
- Establish a process for maintaining an organised approach

The importance of setting priorities

Now that you have had the opportunity to assess your current working practices it is essential that you abandon some of your unproductive habits and start to foster more positive ones.

This chapter aims to support that initiative by introducing you to the concept of setting priorities. If you follow the advice given here you will build some structure into each day and enable yourself to apply much needed focus to the important aspects of your role. Having a sense of order brings with it clarity and enables you to work your way systematically through your commitments. When you understand why you have to accomplish a particular task it makes it easier for you to focus on it. As with anything, when you give a task your full attention because you have committed yourself to it, the chances of it being completed are much higher. Setting priorities greatly reduces the chance of you moving from one job to another in a random and haphazard manner. You will gain a greater sense of achievement and job satisfaction when you review your day and realise you completed everything you had planned.

Priority setting methods

There are a number of methods to choose from, a sample of which are described below. As you will discover, some are more helpful than others, but most of them do not provide the full solution. They are all worth exploring, however, so that you can be clear about their advantages and disadvantages.

Whilst the 80/20 rule will help you in the future to focus on the important parts of your role, you must initially deal with the current situation. You may be feeling overwhelmed at the moment, or do not yet know what you should be focusing on. Perhaps you do not know how to prioritise and continue to react to events that occur during your day rather than applying a systematic approach to your activities.

Doctors favour different approaches, some of which you may be doing already.

Some people favour the "Last in, first out" method. This means that regardless of any original plan or intention, the latest arrival receives instant attention. Some doctors favour this so that their list of things to do does not increase. The usual effect of this approach is that the list does not diminish either, and at the end of the day the best one can hope for is to have maintained the original starting point.

Other doctors prefer the "First in, first out" option. This method sticks to the sequence of delivery and little attention is paid to any looming crises. There is strict adherence to dealing with what came in initially regardless of events that may be occurring in the present. It certainly is one way of prioritising paperwork but it is not the most effective, particularly if the first task or activity bears low significance.

A much favoured option for many doctors is to prioritise the requests of a senior colleague, to whom they report. This method of setting priorities is acceptable as long as the senior colleague is a good time manager. If not, then the situation is worsened. This method also encourages a lack of initiative and proactivity if you fall into the habit of waiting for instructions from above.

Some doctors find themselves responding to the person who shouts the loudest. In a rushed response to make the person go quiet, their work or request is often attended to as a top priority. This system of prioritising cannot be maintained as the response is not based on an accurate assessment of validity or necessity. Attending to someone else's request in order for them to go away and leave you in peace is not the foundation of effective time management. Undertaking your activities in a reactionary way can only encourage you to remain unorganised and unfocused and a victim to the events of the day.

Getting on with the easy tasks as a way of building up to the more complex or important activities is another method of prioritising. However, it is clear to see that this method could be perceived as an escapist activity, an effective way of avoiding what really needs to be done. Whilst you may feel that you have achieved a lot in your day and been very efficient it does not necessarily mean that you have focused on the important things, the activities which add value to your role or objectives. You have simply been busy with undemanding tasks. Following this method could mean that you never attend to the more complex or important issues.

In some professions, the ringing telephone is another favoured method of setting priorities. You may find that you cannot ignore the telephone and no matter what you are dealing with, you leave it in favour of answering the call. As you can see it becomes easy to lose a lot more time than you anticipated. You will often find that the half hour slot you had allocated for a particular task has been reduced to five or ten minutes, due to a telephone call. Frequently the calls lead to further action on your part and your original activity may be abandoned altogether. Do not allow the telephone to dictate your order of priorities.

Do you find yourself drawn to activities or tasks that interest you? Do you favour those at the expense of more mundane activities? If you dislike writing up patient notes, it is likely you will defer doing this and start work on something that you find far more exciting. Notice the energy that accompanies excitement when you embark on something that interests you. It can be tempting to want that feeling for all your duties. However, some things are of a routine nature but are still essential and it is important that you prioritise on that basis rather than your personal enjoyment.

Other methods of setting priorities include starting with the most complex or challenging projects or tasks. Some doctors prefer the opportunity of stretching their intellect or skills, and overlook other tasks in favour of the ones that allow them to gain a strong sense of achievement. Others enjoy such tasks in order to prove to others how highly skilled they are.

What has to be done?

In order to be truly effective and in control there is one method of prioritising that is consistently more successful than any discussed above. If you complete the step by step instructions which follow, you will have begun the important process of self-organisation. Remember that the first part of the process is to deal with the immediate chaos and once you are more organised the same principles can be applied as a long term system for success.

Deal with the present situation

To begin this process, make a list of all outstanding tasks. Write down anything that you know you should have done but, for whatever reason, you have not been able to yet. This is a straightforward list of things to do but now you are going to take the list one step further and actually decide in which order the activities need to be undertaken.

For some doctors, even taking this step can be a revelation. Whilst the limitations of to do lists has already been covered, it is sometimes preferable to not having a list at all. Some doctors prefer not to write anything down and instead, carry a mental list. There are a number of disadvantages with this approach. The brain will continually run a 'stock take' of all outstanding activities and then remind the individual of matters which still require attention. Whilst this could be helpful, the brain does not have a sense of time and will issue reminders at any time during the day or night. This is why some people wake in the middle of the night with a sense of dread at something they have just remembered should have been done but has not. Living in this way is very stressful. Often the list of outstanding jobs feels a lot more when it is held in the mind and many doctors feel burdened by their perceived list of outstanding issues. However, after writing everything down many doctors feel better at seeing the reality of the situation. The brain is no longer burdened and it is able to release the list of outstanding items. Immediately stress levels reduce. In addition, the visible list on paper brings a much stronger sense of reality and frequently the number of items is far less than perceived by the mind. This again is extremely helpful to doctors who are currently overwhelmed and a common reaction is one of relief that things are not as bad as was previously felt or imagined.

Separating important tasks from immediate ones

Once you have your list of everything you need to do, there are only three questions you need to ask of each item:

- Is it essential?

- Does it require my immediate attention?

- If I do not action it, does it have the potential to turn into a crisis?

When deciding if an activity is essential, you need to decide just how serious it is. Should it be at the top of your priorities? When you are organised you will relate this question to your personal objectives. For now, you just need to decide on how serious it is and whether it really is an essential activity that cannot be ignored.

The second question relates to time. How pressing is the activity? Is it something that has to be done today? Consider how you feel about the item. If it feels like it cannot be left for one moment longer then it requires your immediate attention and should be prioritised accordingly.

The third question can be revisited and simply explores the fact that some activities, if left, can turn into a crisis if they are not attended to. Examples of this would be a presentation that you were asked to prepare a month ago. You did not action it because the deadline seemed a long way into the future but now the presentation is tomorrow and you have not started work on it. That work had the potential to turn into a problem if it was not planned and scheduled properly. Some tasks will not have that capacity to change and will not have any impact on you if they are not done until later.

The answer to these questions relies on your judgement and is crucial for good time management. This highly effective approach to setting priorities is based on the time management matrix featured by Dr Stephen Covey in his book, *Seven Habits of Highly Effective People* (2004). This book has adapted these excellent principles and afforded them a medical focus.

Once you have decided how serious your tasks are and whether they require your immediate attention, the next step is to take each activity and move it into the appropriate prioritisation category.

Take 4 sheets of blank A4 paper and do the following, making sure all the sheets are landscape, which means the longer sides are at the top and bottom when you hold them or lay them on the desk in front of you:

On the first piece of paper write the words 'Essential and Immediate' in the middle of the page and draw a circle around them. (An example is given overleaf.)

On the second page write the words, 'Essential but not Immediate' in the middle of the page and draw a circle around the words. On the third page write the words, 'Immediate but not Essential' in the centre and draw a circle around them. On the fourth page write the words, 'Not Immediate and Not Essential' in the middle and draw your circle.

You have now drawn the beginning of 4 mind maps.

A mind map is a diagram used to represent tasks or other items linked to and arranged around a central key word or idea. In relation to managing your time you are going to take each of your outstanding jobs and ask yourself, 'is this task essential and does it require my immediate attention?' When you have your answer, write that task on the relevant mind map sheet.

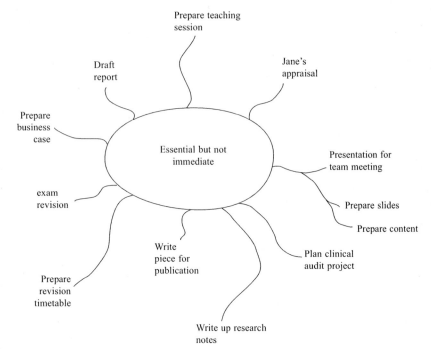

Figure 4.1   Mind map for 'Essential but not Immediate' tasks

When this exercise is complete, you will have allocated all your outstanding tasks to one of the four mind maps.

It will be obvious to you that any tasks you have allocated to the 'essential and immediate' mind map are those that must be started immediately. These are tasks with overdue deadlines or imminent ones and create that sense of urgency or even panic when you think about them. They could constitute a crisis for you and please be clear that these activities are not ones that you can delegate. Examples of 'essential and immediate' items might be formal complaints from patients, overdue work, crises that require a reactionary approach and large tasks with impending deadlines. They literally must be done either today or within the next few days because you have ignored them for too long. Sometimes doctors consider everything to be a crisis if it does not receive immediate attention, but in reality this is rarely the case. Take a disciplined look at only the jobs you have not yet done and be realistic about each one. Concentrate on the activities that you know you cannot put off until tomorrow. Do not worry about unforeseen events that may impact upon you, because you will continue to procrastinate and worry. Effective time managers take action and with decisiveness. Start to solve the immediate issue and deal with each crisis activity.

Many doctors find, with some relief, that many of their outstanding and stressful items are indeed essential, i.e. extremely important, but do not require immediate attention. This is good news because straight away the opportunity has arisen to plan ahead. You will find many activities can be planned and scheduled in an organised manner, because you now have a clear sense that they are not 'immediate' tasks and can wait. However, you will still acknowledge the fact that they are essential tasks which have to be carried out at some point in the future. Please note that the 'essential but not immediate' mind map should require a bigger sheet of paper and that is a great position in which to find yourself. The more of your actions are assigned to this mind map, the better the situation for you.

Examples of items that can be planned will be activities such as clinical research, building relationships with colleagues, preparation for presentations, thinking strategically, writing for publication, clinical audit and conducting a staff appraisal. When you become organised you will find that this mind map will always have a lot more in it than the other categories and so it should. This is where all of your planning takes place and your overall intention should be to spend most of your time in this area.

The examples of activities given in this chapter are generalisations because for each doctor the outstanding items will be different. The examples provided are just to give you an idea of the sorts of things that may be on your list. As you are discovering already, your judgement will be subjective and you must decide what is essential for you and what must be done today.

You may also find some tasks which are not essential but seemingly require immediate attention. This is the category most likely to cause confusion. Many doctors who struggle to manage their time properly misinterpret the immediate element as being urgent and place it on the 'essential and immediate' mind map when it does not actually belong there. These tasks or actions are not essential for you and will not impact positively on your day. However, they may be essential for someone else and they are certainly desired by someone else to be done today or this week. That may be true for the other person but what you must be clear about is that it is not down to you to make that task a priority. These requests often come your way when the person responsible for the task is also having difficulties with their time management. They try and make their crisis your crisis and pressurise you into acting quickly so that their work can be done on time. Resist these people. Being clear about your own priorities will help you to do so. Examples of 'not essential but immediate' actions could be a request from someone else to sort out their problem which has little or nothing to do with you. Some meetings and e-mails will fall into this category, as will requests from other people to do them a favour. Apparent emergencies constitute 'not essential but immediate' items and frequently involve a senior colleague. Think rationally and do not allow yourself to react to the shouting. Ask yourself the key questions – is this essential for me, even though I know it is for my senior, and does it require my immediate attention? In most cases the answer is no, so please ask the question before rushing to give into the demands of others. Challenge these requests and find out just how serious and timely the issue is. When questioned, the requester will often revise his or her position and may even re-evaluate the situation and back down.

The final category is reserved for those items which are 'not essential and not immediate' so they are of minimal or no importance and have no urgency attached to them. Anything that you regard as trivial should be allocated to this mind map. Items which constitute comfort or escapist activities are ideal for placing here in your list of priorities. Not only should they appear last in your order of priorities, one might argue that they should not appear at all. Computer games, junk e-mails, excessive cigarette and coffee breaks, gossip and reading irrelevant material are ways of wasting time and should be curtailed or stopped altogether.

Unfortunately for some people, these trivial activities provide a welcome antidote to the crisis management method they habitually adopt. Individuals who spend the majority of their day involved with adrenalin-fuelled activities will lose themselves in escapist activities, from time to time during the day, just to get a break. This way of working is unsustainable over the long term, not just for the individual concerned but for everyone who is impacted by his or her actions. It is probable that you will not have many activities on this mind map, but be very honest, in case you have developed a coffee habit which could benefit from being reduced.

Categorising your outstanding activities in this manner is a fantastic way of dealing with the current situation. Now you have a clear picture of where to begin and where to focus your energy and determination. Deal with all essential tasks that must be attended to immediately. Only when you have done this will you feel able to start organising your time and activities for the future, with the aim being to avoid a similar situation from happening again. It is always a choice and the decision to do things differently can only lie with you but if you really want to become an effective and well respected doctor it is worth trying an alternative approach to self-organisation.

Your long term aim is to approach all your responsibilities in this way. Once you have organised your immediate tasks into the correct order based upon the essential and time-framed criteria, you will eventually deal with future requests for your time with the same perspective. Once you can demonstrate to others how you prioritise your work they will start to work with you. As you begin to influence and educate those around you, their approach to time management and organisation may change to reflect your practices more closely. As an ongoing process, be prepared to update your priorities as the longer term projects will often change in status. Revisit each one and double check that the priority remains the same.

When faced with a demand for immediate action, as no doubt you will be, apply the same criteria that you would for your own planned activities. Find out how essential the work is and whether it is a priority for today. If it is, discuss with the requester your other 'essential and immediate' activities and agree together which ones you will drop in order to make room for the additional work. This provides a useful test of the original request. The other person may not have realised how busy you are and will retract the request or, they will agree to take responsibility for some other planned activity not being done. This does happen and is acceptable if you have reached this decision by mutual agreement.

If it is not appropriate to discuss your planned activities with another person then make the decision for yourself. If you feel you need to undertake the request then decide which of your scheduled tasks for that day you can realistically drop and ensure that you plan it into another day.

Having taken the trouble to organise your current outstanding tasks, have the confidence to focus on them to the exclusion of everything else until the immediate crises are out of the way. By agreeing to take on more and more work within impossible deadlines only leads to ineffectiveness and stress. So be firm and be reasonable with people, but do focus on what matters most: your priorities.

The next two chapters will show you how to deal with the situation now that you are fully aware of it and, help you foster a positive habit of organising your activities each week.

Exercise

If you have not done so already, list all outstanding tasks, however large or small.

Consider each action in turn and ask yourself:

- Is this task essential (i.e. is it highly significant?)

- Does this task require my immediate attention? (Gauge your instincts; should you be dealing with this today or tomorrow?)

Take 4 sheets of A4 paper and create mind maps for each category.

The categories are:

ESSENTIAL AND IMMEDIATE

ESSENTIAL BUT NOT IMMEDIATE

IMMEDIATE BUT NOT ESSENTIAL

NOT ESSENTIAL AND NOT IMMEDIATE

Every one of your actions must be assigned to one of the above mind maps. Do not allocate according to unfounded fears of what might happen. Look at each task as it stands today and ascertain for yourself whether you should be taking that action today or whether it is, in fact, an escapist activity which should be assigned to the fourth mind map.

Once you have done this, re-visit the items in the ESSENTIAL BUT NOT IMMEDIATE mind map and consider what will happen if you do not action them. This will help create a sub-priority system within the ESSENTIAL BUT NOT IMMEDIATE category for those items which have the potential to turn into a crisis.

Once all actions are assigned you are now in a position to deal with each one in a defined order of priority and regain control of your workload.

Summary

- Before you can adopt planning strategies you must deal with the current situation.

- An effective way of breaking the chaotic cycle is to prioritise all outstanding items.

- Making a list of outstanding things to do may help reduce stress levels simply by allowing your mind to let go of all your outstanding actions.

- You may find that there is less to do than you thought.

- Prioritising your To-Do list helps you understand where to apply your energy.

- Using the Essential/Immediate criteria helps you determine what must be done first.

- Once you have a system for prioritising, this can be applied to all future activities.

- Having a priority system allows you to demonstrate your organised approach to others.

- Discuss with them the urgency and importance of their request.

- If necessary, agree with the other party the activities which you will drop in order to fit their request into your schedule.

- Do not agree to additional requests until your 'essential and immediate' items are cleared.

References

Stephen Covey, *The 7 Habits of Highly Effective People* Simon and Schuster UK Ltd (2004)

Chapter 5   Dealing with the situation

Aims & objectives

In this chapter you will:

- Understand why taking action is key to successful time management
- Start work on your highest priority work
- Deal with non-essential but urgent work
- Develop a strategy to handle escapist activities
- Develop the positive habit of planning future tasks and responsibilities
- Cultivate the positive habit of planning your workload on a weekly basis

The importance of taking action

If you completed the exercise in the last chapter you will have successfully arranged your tasks into an order of priorities and be in a great position to deal with the most urgent. However daunting your mind maps are, it is much better for you to understand the reality of your situation. With clarity comes focus and you should now be able to give your attention easily to the tasks which require it the most. For some of you the 'essential and immediate'mind map may contain far fewer items than you anticipated and you will be experiencing some relief at this. For others of you the reality will be just as bad as you feared and you will find yourself with a number of essential and immediate activities which require instant action from you.

Whatever your position, it is time to start actioning your priority mind maps.

Your highest priority

The mind map of tasks which requires your immediate attention is the first one – 'essential and immediate'. These are the tasks which you cannot ignore any longer. These items cannot be delegated to others and must be done by you. Do not waste your energy feeling sorry for yourself or allowing your stress levels to increase. Successful time managers understand that the only way out of chaos is to take action. So, re-examine your mind map of 'essential and immediate' items and decide which one you can realistically begin with. Try and organise this category into another set of priorities. All of these activities obviously take precedence over everything else but it will help you move forward if you organise this sub-category into some kind of order. Which item must you attend to before all others? You may find a few undertakings that you would class as a must, in which case group these together on your mind map. You may want to mark them with a 'TP' for Top Priority or 'M' for Must. Do whatever works for you but do this quickly. You cannot put these off any longer and do not allow this sub-prioritisation to become another way to procrastinate. You must act and get them done.

The benefit of these mind maps is that they allow you to organise yourself and gain a much clearer idea of what needs to be done. However, it is still up to you to find your motivation and get on with the tasks.

Return to your mind map and decide which of the items on your 'essential and immediate' category should be done next. Mark these items with an 'S' for Should or choose a label which is meaningful for you. Whatever is left will be the last things that you do on your essential list.

It is to be hoped that there are not too many items in the top priority category. You may have already found that using this method of prioritising has given you a greater sense of control, even before you have started to address your tasks. This is because, psychologically, the burden of outstanding activities often feels worse than the reality. If nothing else, discovering that there are very few activities which actually do have to be done today, or imminently, can be the perfect motivation to getting started. Those feelings of being overwhelmed are dissipated and confidence in your ability to get through your workload returns. This may be all the motivation you need.

So what happens now? The first thing you must do is deal with the situation in which you find yourself. Open your diary for the coming week and schedule some of your 'essential and immediate' tasks. It will be a matter of judgement regarding how many you can complete in one week and if you are unsure, err on the side of caution. It is advisable to schedule one or two items a week, to begin with, particularly if you are not sure how long each job will take.

If you do not have many tasks that require your immediate attention, you may be in the fortunate position of being able to schedule all of them into your diary for this week. Whatever the case, start scheduling for the coming week and give yourself enough time to achieve each one.

If you are still feeling overwhelmed, then select just one item that you have marked as 'TP'. Getting one thing done is better than nothing but make the commitment to yourself to achieve that one thing. Imagine the satisfaction of crossing it off your mind map once it is complete!

Dealing with the unessential

If you find the majority of your outstanding activities are in the second category of 'essential but not immediate', then congratulations! At last you have the opportunity to become organised, focused and plan your future activities. How you start to deal with 'essential but not immediate' items will be covered a little later in this chapter.

Dealing with the unimportant

Take a look at what you have allocated to the third category. This referred to tasks which you decided were 'not essential but immediate' items. As stated in the previous chapter, this is a potentially confusing category for some but it need not be. This predominantly relates to tasks which are important or imminent for other people. The key factor to remember with this category is the 'not essential' part. Instead of focusing on the urgency, which may tempt you to make it your priority, you have to be clear about whether the task is actually important to you in the context of your role, or your objectives. Usually these jobs are not essential to you, or for you. You will not benefit by doing this work, even if someone else has asked you to do it. You have already made the decision about the tasks' significance in your working life and by allocating them to the third category of priorities, it is clear that you are aware of their low impact.

When you become organised and are in the enviable position of dealing with only future work, you will easily know what to do with the items that fall into the 'not essential but immediate' category. You will have established that this work will not help you achieve your objectives and does not constitute a top priority for you. Therefore, you will either refuse it or get someone else to do it. If you feel you must accept it, it should be one of the last things you schedule into your weekly activities.

As you are still in the process of becoming organised, it is likely that you may have agreed to some work which falls into this category. Unfortunately, as with the higher priority items, now that you have accepted it, you must find a way of dealing with it.

If you can, the best option for you is to find someone else to whom you can delegate. If you distract yourself with work that does not form part of your top priorities it will, of course, keep you from doing the work you should be focusing on. You will continue to work in a somewhat reactive way and your efforts at becoming more organised will be undermined. If you feel you are not in a position to delegate or have no-one to whom you can delegate, ask your peer colleagues if they can help you. Or discuss your situation with the person that gave you the work in the first place and see if they can find someone else. If all else fails you will have to do the work yourself but make sure you do it in the order of priority you have set. You must deal with the highly 'essential and immediate' tasks first and include some actions from the second highest priority category: those items which are 'essential but not immediate'. Only then should you be thinking about undertaking someone else's work or request. Be clear: the work that you assign to the 'not essential but immediate' category should really be done by someone other than you. You cannot afford to be distracted. Delegation is a difficult proficiency for some doctors but it forms part of the competencies outlined within *The Medical Leadership Competency Framework* and is a key management skill. It is critical that you perfect this skill as it will serve you well in your medical career and achieve significant improvements in your time management.

Strategies for dealing with escapism

You probably realise by now that anything in the last category, 'not essential and not immediate, should not receive your attention at all. Most items assigned to this fourth priority can be described as trivial activities and have no positive impact on your objectives. They serve as a means of escape from the stress-ridden approach of 'essential and immediate' items but should not be actioned at all during the working day. Junk emails and social networking websites are electronic forms of escapism. Make an effort to ignore them. Non-clinical publications should be left until your commitments are achieved, or perhaps when you travel home and want to unwind on the train. It is to be hoped that you will now be so focused, working through your scheduled priorities, that you will not have time for trivia. When you are more organised, you will be planning your weekly diary around your second mind map. As a result you will approach your work in a much more calm and controlled manner and no longer experience the anxiety of thinking about work responsibilities that have not been met. As your stress levels reduce, so should your need to lose yourself in a meaningless and time-stealing activity. Do not forget that escapist habits are hard to break and at first it will need a determined effort from you. Do persevere because there are plenty of more important things for you to be doing.

Planning the important things

Ideally, the second mind map of 'essential but not immediate' is where you need to be placing your attention. Understanding the importance of certain tasks but realising that they do not all have to be done immediately puts you in the best place to become organised. For many doctors, a lot of outstanding activities will fall into this category. This is good news because it allows you to schedule them into your diary in a planned and controlled manner. If you are to become effective in your time management, then you must nurture a positive habit of dealing with your 'essential but not immediate' tasks and not put them off. Otherwise they may turn into a crisis and you are back to square one. Get into the habit of scheduling a manageable amount of work, one that does not overwhelm you or decrease your motivation.

If you have not got many crisis tasks then you may want to schedule some actions from the 'essential but not immediate' mind map right away. In the long term, when you are organised, you will schedule some activities from your second mind map every week. This means you will steadily work your way through the tasks which are most important to you and become experienced at judging how long things will take to get done. Even the projects which have distant deadlines can be commenced now, so that when the target date approaches, you will have achieved most of the work, week by week, in manageable chunks.

There will be many tangible activities that are easy to schedule but consider all the other responsibilities associated with your role. Some of you will need to build in time to think. This may strike you as odd but not enough time is set aside for thinking things through. Many communications and relationships would benefit from a more measured and thought out approach. All too often, face to face interactions or rushed emails create the wrong impression and may damage a necessary relationship. Major projects require thinking time as part of preparation, as do the creation of presentations and reports. Senior doctors will require strategic thinking time where they can start to shape the future of their service. They also need to consider the strategies that will need to be implemented in order to fulfil their vision of the future.

The importance of a weekly routine

The advice throughout this chapter has been to schedule your tasks on a weekly basis. What is so significant about this? Attempting to plan your workload on a day by day basis does not progress you from making a 'to do' list. You may continue to feel anxious and have that sense of urgency. Conversely, when you have sight of the whole week ahead, you have a far greater sense of perspective and control. As said before, you are in a much better position to plan. Even interruptions and unexpected events can be given room.

Spread out your tasks so that you do not overwhelm one day with too much to do. Ensure that all your fixed and regular commitments are also in your diary. Include your clinics, ward rounds, team meetings and any other regularly occurring activity. You need a clear picture of your weekly commitments before you can make additions. Pace yourself and be realistic about what you can achieve. After all your regular commitments are on paper in front of you or on a computer screen in electronic format, you will be able to identify gaps in each day. Schedule your outstanding and highest priority tasks into the gaps, ensuring that there is enough time to deal with them or at least make a major impact on a large undertaking.

At this stage you are trying to get back on track and your focus must be aimed at clearing the backlog of work. Give yourself one month to clear the build up and each Monday repeat the above exercise, carefully scheduling your top priority tasks into the gaps in your schedule. This is a great habit to practise and as most new habits take a month to become natural, the four-week deadline suits both purposes. If you make a commitment to try this method of transferring your priorities to your diary each week, it is hoped that you will have enough motivation to actually complete them. If you find yourself slipping then reduce the number of 'essential and immediate' and 'essential but not immediate' items in your working week. Very quickly you will clear the mind map of top priority issues as you will have focused on these exclusively to begin with. Now you can move to your 'essential but not immediate' items and get a real sense of organisation. As you progress with these you will increase your productivity, reduce your stress levels and gain in confidence. Other people will also notice a change in you and how much calmer or happier you appear and this positive cycle becomes self-perpetuating.

If you have delegated as much of the 'not essential but immediate' items to other people, you can start to focus on the key mind map of tasks which are important to you but do not have to be actioned immediately. Once you have caught up, there is no reason to stop prioritising and planning and every reason to continue. Make this your positive habit and maintain your commitment to becoming an effective time manager.

Your mission is to maintain the status quo and consider every request or responsibility with new eyes. Ask the same key questions of each piece of work. Is it essential? Does it have to be done today? Maintain your mind maps so that you always have a picture of your workload. Schedule some tasks from 'essential but not immediate' each week so that you always progress and action your priorities which can only move you closer to the achievement of your objectives.

Doctors are continually interrupted and report that many unexpected events occur during their week. This is no reason to be pulled back into chaotic working practices. Now that you have established a great system for dealing with your work, all you need to do is preserve some gaps in the day. Do not cram too many activities into each day so that you cannot manage it all. Good time management will never prevent unexpected events, due to their very nature, but it will enable you to deal with them without stress. You may have to re-schedule certain planned items in the day but you will have space in the diary to do so. This approach keeps you firmly in control and your ability to cope with the unexpected is undiminished. Once you get used to this new system of working you can also plan for interruptions. Using the same logic, leave some time free each day so that you have made provision for interruptions should they happen. You may consider having some small tasks on stand-by in case you find yourself with some spare time. This would be highly proactive and would ensure that you continue to use your time productively. If you are a senior doctor who allows junior staff to interrupt with queries during times you have allocated for high priority commitments, consider scheduling a regular face to face meeting once a week with each member of the team. Perhaps if they know they will have the opportunity to spend some official time with you they will stop interrupting you when you have more important tasks to deal with.

As you can see, it is one thing to schedule the task in your diary, but quite another to ensure that you actually get on with it. Not only must you make the time, but you must also protect it. Having allocated some time to do a specific task, do not allow yourself to be interrupted or distracted. Close the door, take the phone off the hook or find a quite place. Do whatever it takes but be committed to getting the job done. Having got yourself out of trouble, do not let old habits creep back in. Protect the time you have allocated and focus on the task in hand.

Exercise

Look at the week ahead in your diary or electronic calendar and ensure that all your regular commitments are scheduled in. Leave nothing out. You must have a clear picture of your fixed and regular workload.

Identify the gaps in each day and schedule as many of your top priority tasks as possible, taking care not to put in too many at first. You have to work out your limits and capacity for getting things done. You may overwhelm yourself with too many tasks at once, so begin slowly, but be determined to complete the few that you do schedule.

If you have a lot of outstanding things to do in the 'essential and immediate' category, focus only on these. If you have very few or none at all, introduce one or two tasks each week from your 'essential but not immediate' mind-map or category.

Start with this week and schedule some tasks now. Leave some gaps each day. This may mean, on a particularly busy day, that you are unable to schedule an outstanding task. This is okay. It is better to be realistic. Starting with only one or two tasks over the week should enable you to make progress. As you gain in confidence you will be able to complete more tasks each week.

Repeat this exercise every week for four weeks. Cross off each task as you complete it, from your mind map or box. Focus only on the top two priority categories. Delegate or abandon the rest of your outstanding tasks.

Summary

- Having identified and arranged your priorities, it is important to deal with the situation.

- Start to schedule your 'essential and immediate' items straight away.

- You must delegate 'not essential but immediate' items which are important or urgent for other people but not for you.

- Having worked out your tasks into an order of priority you must now move them into your diary and make a commitment to action them.

- Established priorities must be transferred into the diary on a week by week basis.

- Ensure all your regular clinical and non-clinical commitments are in the diary already.

- When you have resolved the current situation you will be organised and in control.

- You will approach all future work in the same logical and structured way.

- You will be able to plan all future actions.

- You will diarise one or two actions to begin with each week until you get used to completing what you intended.

- Ensure that you always leave gaps in your working day to allow for interruptions and unexpected events. You know they will happen, you just don't know when, so plan for them.

Chapter 6 Time for reflection

Aims & objectives

In this chapter you will:

- Reflect on your behaviour and beliefs that allow these situations to arise

- Deal with your resistance to change and coach yourself for improved performance

Hopefully you have either started, or are considering starting, a new way of organising your time, based on priorities. This strategy will undoubtedly get you out of the chaos you may be experiencing in your current situation. Soon you will be ready to maintain this habit and organise all future work commitments in a similar way. Before you do that it is worth taking a moment to pause and reflect on how you have got yourself into this situation in the first place. You will see from the amount of tasks in each mind map what influences you or perhaps whom. You should be able to gain useful insights into your working practices and this chapter enables you to explore the reasons why you have chosen to work in this way. When faced with your bad habits you may feel resistant to change and come up with a number of explanations. You may feel defensive or frustrated if you believe nothing can change. Do remember that you have a choice and it is not this way for everyone. Some people are able to manage the requests and interruptions during their working day and still achieve what they had planned. If it is possible for them, it is possible for you, if you are willing.

This chapter explores your resistance to moving away from a crisis or reactionary mindset. It will also mention potential resistance to delegating and saying no to other people, particularly the person to whom you report. However, as these are significant factors in successful time management, they are covered in greater detail in separate chapters. Some doctors resist the boredom of having every activity planned. It is important that you consider your reasons for resisting the change and then develop effective strategies to overcome them. This is a short chapter, simply designed to help you work out any inner conflict that arises when you consider implementing new strategies.

It serves as a useful place in which to pause and reflect on your personal style and to explore your unconscious motivations that have caused you to become disorganised.

Begin with the crisis category. How many items do you have in the 'essential and immediate' section? Is it every bit as bad as you thought it was going to be? If it is then you need to resolve this situation as soon as possible. There is no way around it. This is not effective time management and must be the first category to address if you are going to see the improvements you wish.

As this chapter is devoted to self-reflection, ask yourself why you have allowed this situation to develop? What are your reasons for allowing things to build up until they become a crisis with an imminent deadline?

Some doctors enjoy working in an adrenaline-fuelled environment. They thrive on the pace of running from one situation to another, just meeting their deadlines and handling the crises as they arise. For some doctors this affords them the opportunity to demonstrate how capable they are. They like the idea that they are perceived as the one who saves the day or can always be relied upon in a crisis. Whilst these are undoubtedly useful traits in an emergency situation, they do not make for effective time management. Which reasons apply to you? Does rushing from one event to another, in order to meet last minute deadlines make you feel more powerful or capable? Or are you aware of other reasons why you put things off? Be very honest and try and find the answer to why you do not deal with things until they become a crisis. This does not refer to unexpected events. It relates specifically to tasks which you did have plenty of time to do, or plenty of notice, but for whatever reason, you neglected.

Some doctors put off doing certain tasks for the reasons outlined in chapter two. Do you let things slide because you resist them? Do you put projects or presentations off because they seem too daunting or require too much effort? This happens to many doctors who struggle to organise themselves effectively but remember that good time managers take action. Once a project has begun it becomes far easier to manage, both psychologically and physically. Remember that when you procrastinate you actually increase your feelings of stress, not diminish them. The burden will not leave you until the project has been started.

It is important for you to understand your habits or motivations for being in this situation so that you can work out an action plan for change.

Take some time now to coach yourself about your performance. Fill in each box in table 6.1.

What has to change in order for me to reduce the amount of tasks in the 'essential and immediate' category?	
How can I persuade myself to deal with tasks sooner?	

Table 6.1   Interactive Chart for performance self-analysis

Why do I need the adrenaline rush that dealing with a crisis gives me?	
What am I trying to demonstrate about myself to other people?	
How could I demonstrate the same qualities or skills in a more productive way?	
How can I overcome my resistance to certain tasks or projects?	
What are the benefits of me being more proactive when the project has a distant deadline?	
What would be the benefits of feeling less stressed?	
What immediate steps can I take, in relation to time, to reduce my stress?	

Table 6.1   Continued

No-one else has to see your answers. This is just for you and serves as your chance for total scrutiny and honesty. This is part of nurturing your commitment to change in favour of better time management practices.

Now look at the 'not essential but immediate' category. This is the area which should be delegated completely. Remember that these items are with you as a result of other people not managing their time properly. Consider your resistance to delegating. What stops you? Some doctors feel that they should not delegate. They fear they are passing on their burden to someone else. You cannot afford to feel this way. It will become clear to you that you should not have agreed to take on the work in the first place but now that you have it is better for you to delegate it so that it can be done, while allowing you to focus on your higher priority work.

Some doctors feel guilty for giving some of their work away and others find it impossible to say no to the requests of someone senior. Some do not even feel able to ask for help from a colleague.

If the work has been delegated to you from a senior colleague it may be true that you cannot ask someone else to do it. However, it will still be up to you to decide upon its priority in your workload. Do not deviate from your new habit of prioritising and scheduling. Treat this request like any other. As looked at previously, some doctors view any work handed down from above to be of the highest priority. It would be advisable for you to find out before making this assumption. This book is not suggesting that you refuse to do work given to you by your senior, but it does advocate investigating how urgent it is. Your senior may surprise you and inform you that it does not need to be done immediately in which case you can prioritise it accordingly and schedule it in behind other tasks.

Consider agreeing a deadline with your senior. There is often room for negotiation but our assumptions prevent us from speaking up. Now that you are taking ownership of your personal effectiveness you will need to take a proactive approach. It is an easy thing to do and yet avoided by so many. Although there is a strong hierarchy within medicine, do not let that disrupt your organisation. It will be your judgement ultimately, but most senior colleagues would not take offence at being asked how quickly the task they have delegated needs to be done.

Many doctors are adamant that their seniors cannot be questioned in any way and their instructions must be carried out immediately but this is simply not the case. However, it is true to say that anyone who is unchallenged will often not offer an alternative. In other words they will let you run around, putting their work ahead of yours, as long as you allow them to. Consider the possibility of discussing your workload with them and agreeing with them when you will be able to carry out their request.

If they then insist that their work has to be done now, at least you have found out and received clear confirmation.

If you still feel resistant to this approach, ask yourself why. What is it about directly communicating with your senior that troubles you? Why do you feel that work delegated to you automatically falls into the 'essential and immediate' mind map? What stops you from finding out?

If you are in a senior position you may dislike delegating to junior staff. The same rules apply. You have more important things to be getting on with and anything that you have allocated to your 'not essential but immediate' section must be given to other people. The motivation to do so may lie in the understanding that you have a responsibility to develop your team. A forthcoming chapter will cover the process of delegating in full, which may alleviate some doubt or confusion about what can or cannot be delegated. Perhaps you do not know how to delegate. This chapter is more concerned with why you do not want to or what stops you. Take time now to reflect on this and write down all your reasons for resisting this course of action.

Examine your answers and think about how to overcome your resistance. What are the consequences of you not improving your time management? Just as you questioned yourself about moving away from crisis management, do the same with 'not essential but immediate' items. Be clear about why you do not want to delegate and what feelings you experience when you think about it.

Here are some useful questions with which you can coach yourself:

What are the consequences of not developing your juniors?	
How will that affect their training?	

Table 6.2   Self Analysis

How motivated will they be if they perceive that you do not trust them enough to delegate some of your work?	
What is the cost to you?	
What is the impact on your higher priority tasks if you cannot delegate unimportant pieces of work to other people?	

Table 6.2   Continued

Be honest and tough on yourself. Something has to shift in your belief system or you are never going to become effective at managing your time. At least be courageous enough to try.

It is imperative that you raise your awareness of your thoughts and feelings because if they remain unconscious then you are prevented from dealing with them, and yet they could be working against you and holding you back.

To complete your self-reflection, answer the final set of coaching questions:

What stops me from talking to my seniors about work they have given me?	
How could I approach them in a non-confrontational way?	

Table 6.3   Self coaching questions

What deadline would I like to agree?	
What other questions do I need to ask?	
What would be a useful compromise?	
Why am I afraid to communicate with them?	
Why do I assume this conversation will be confrontational?	
If I do not, what stops me?	
What unconscious assumptions do I make?	
What will be the impact on my career if I do not learn to delegate?	

Table 6.3   Continued

What is my reputation with regards to time management?	
How can I improve it?	
What small steps can I take today that will make a difference?	
What perception of myself do I want to create in others?	
How can I achieve this?	

Table 6.3   Continued

Exercise

Examine the areas of crisis management, delegation and saying no and note the one that you resist the most. Refer back to the answers you gave to the coaching questions and consider what you need to do in order to overcome your natural resistance.

As this is an exercise in self-reflection, be honest and write down your reasons for not wanting to change. Note your thoughts and feelings.

Be open to the possibilities of alternative options and now write down statements of intent, detailing what you are going to do to help you push through your self-imposed barriers or limiting beliefs.

Put together a detailed action plan, outlining the steps you will take.

Summary

- It is important to reflect on working practices in order to discover unconscious beliefs or responses which have given rise to the existing situation.

- It can be difficult to accept that fighting one crisis after another does not have to be the only way to function in medicine.

- Regaining control of how you spend your time is only possible when you relinquish this habit.

- When accepting work from a senior colleague, find out the true deadline.

- It is unhelpful to make assumptions about the deadline for delegated work

- Self-reflection is a useful way of discovering unconscious motivations for behaviour.

- Action plans provide proactive strategies for overcoming resistance to change.

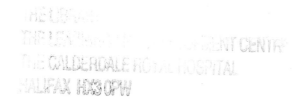

Chapter 7 Time to focus

Aims & objectives

In this chapter you will:

- Discover the secrets of effective time managers
- Understand how focus is the key to long term organisation
- Develop strategies to help maintain your focus
- Understand the importance of goals and objectives
- Be able to create measurable objectives to increase your motivation
- Start looking at the bigger picture of your life
- Realise the importance of taking action, however small
- Apply the five minute rule to tasks you put off

Having used the mind maps to re-establish a sense of order to your existing obligations and reflected upon the changes you need to make to prevent the situation from re-occurring, it is important that you develop some practical strategies. However, this seems easier said than done for most people, no matter what their profession. It is undoubtedly a real challenge for doctors who have many demands placed upon them. However, having identified your priorities and started to extract yourself from a chaotic situation, it is just as important for you to learn new strategies that will keep you working in an organised and proactive manner. As this book has revealed, a lack of focus is often the obstacle to effective time management. When surrounded by patient requirements for time and attention, colleagues wanting your help, seniors needing to delegate to you, in addition to a number of things that you have not yet gotten around to, it can become difficult to deal with anything at all. It is far more likely that you will feel overwhelmed and seek refuge in escapist activities, meaningless ways of spending your time which may make you feel better but are not helpful to you in the long run.

This chapter aims to show you how to develop that focus so that you can put strategies in place which will help you stay organised. Setting priorities each week is one useful method and this chapter explores the benefits of having objectives as a means of providing long term motivation for self-organisation.

Good time management initiatives

This chapter hopes to offer you techniques and tips that will help you gain some focus and understanding about what is important to you and what you should be spending your time on. It aims to help you become effective in getting the right things done in the right amount of time. It may be helpful for you to know what you're aiming for so this chapter begins by revealing the initiatives of successful doctors who manage their time well. Understanding their approach may help you identify areas that you need to develop.

The first initiative is to be able to view your activities within the wider context of work-related objectives or even life goals. Once you have a strong sense of purpose, you can direct any activities towards fulfilling that purpose. Without purpose, you run the risk of being side-tracked by more trivial tasks, simply because you do not have a clear idea of what you should be concentrating on. You may be guilty of being very busy and fooling yourself that you are efficient, but what will you have achieved that could be described as effective?

The second initiative is to become more decisive. The quicker you can make decisions the easier it will be for you to get things done. This is common sense but often proves to be problematical for many. Once you have developed the habit of making firm decisions in a timely way you can then start acting on those decisions. If you are currently allowing yourself to be distracted by other things or other people it is because you have either not yet made a decision to do something or you have not stuck to the decision. Get into the positive habit of acting upon your decisions once you have made them. The third initiative is determination. A doctor who is successful at time management will decide to do something and will not allow distraction. Think about your role models in medicine. Having decided to embark upon a job, did they focus their attention on that one undertaking and not stop until they had completed it? If you are not like your role model, it is likely you are unable to maintain your focus or determination and allow yourself to be sidetracked by other matters. All this does is increase your stress levels as you feel out of control and realise that yet another job has not been finished and will have to be attended to another day.

The fourth initiative concerns taking action. Everyone encounters tasks or projects that they fear or feel apprehensive about. Doctors who struggle the most with time management react to this emotion by avoiding the undertaking. They believe that by deferring it for as long as possible they will feel less worried or that the job will disappear altogether. Remember the advice given in Chapter Two which states that the opposite is usually true. Understand that the best way to overcome reluctance or fear of a task is to get on with it. Overcome your doubt with action.

Taking action, however small, is better than doing nothing at all. Stress levels do diminish once a project or activity is started and it often proves to be much less daunting than it appeared. Doctors who manage their time effectively are proactive and have got on with tasks. They have not put things off until the last minute and have been able to accomplish much more of their work in a controlled and steady manner.

The fifth and final element of success involves having systems to deal with paperwork, telephone calls and interruptions. Creating these systems enables you to leave on time if you choose, with a clear desk and peace of mind. Doctors who do not have systems leave themselves vulnerable to increasing workloads that they do not know how to manage. You need to know what to do with every bit of paper that crosses your desk. You need to develop a strategy that enables you to deal with that paperwork, instead of pushing it around on your desk or continually creating piles of paper to be dealt with at an unspecified future date. Dealing with things is the only way to become successful at organising yourself and managing your stress. Chapter Eleven will show you how to develop such systems.

Focus is the key to long-term organisation

It is evident that the first step to becoming organised is developing focus. You may find that identifying your priorities, through the mind maps, provides you with just the focus you need. However, some of you might also like to implement the 80/20 rule, as described in Chapter Three. As you now realise, as little as twenty per cent of your work will produce eighty per cent of your results. This means that only twenty per cent of your time will deal with productive activities. Less productive activities include reading e-mails, taking telephone calls and attending some meetings that do not affect you or where you have limited influence. The twenty per cent will yield high value results and may include essential decisions about patient care or improvements to the service you provide. It may concern a decision about procuring a new piece of equipment, or putting together a business case for extra funding. For some doctors the 80/20 rule may be more relevant around colleagues. You may encounter colleagues who take up the majority of your time but give little in return. So how can you apply the 80/20 rule at work? How much time are you able to devote to the most productive activities in your week? Doctors have reported, anecdotally, that they spend less than twenty per cent of their time on the most productive tasks. Are you doing the same?

Time management tip

Identify your top yielding 20 percent of activities and do more of them.

If you feel you need more focus than prioritising gives you, make a list of the ten things that occupy most of your time at work. Do not produce a job description of what you should be doing. Be honest and detail the reality. This is not quite the same as keeping a detailed time log which can help you identify the interruptions and time wasters. This is more of an overview of your general activities, trying to help you identify which ones yield the most value and which the least. Against each activity assign a percentage. This is your estimate of how long you spend on that activity. For example:

1.   Recording patient information (10%)

2.   Reading e-mails (15%)

3.   Attending meetings (40%)

4.   Ward rounds (25%)

Keep going until you reach ten activities. It does not really matter whether they exceed a hundred percent of your time. It is more important to work out how valuable each activity is. Once you have got a complete list, detail the three items that add the most value in your opinion.

Estimate how much time you spend on your top three. Your goal will be to start spending much more time on these high yielding activities. Many doctors feel that this is an unrealistic approach because there is simply too much to do. However, that is rarely the case. It is much more linked to the inability to say no to other people and the lack of awareness which makes it difficult to know which activities should be focused on. By identifying your high yielding activities you will develop strategies to deal with the low yielding eighty percent of your work. You will be able to delegate or decline further requests to take on extra responsibilities. Or you will defer some activities to a later date when you are able to plan them into your schedule.

Maintaining your focus

It is clear to see that effective time managers are in control of their lives. In order for you to be a successful doctor you need to take control of your life too. The fundamental way to begin this process is to know what you want. Setting goals and objectives is a critical strategy for developing focus and motivation. It is a fantastic way of deciding what you should be dealing with and what should be left. Once you have set some goals or objectives and have something to aim for, you should only undertake those tasks which will help you reach them. Having a clear idea about what you want from life prevents you giving in to the demands of others and maintaining destructive habits that do not add value to your life. Having an end result in your mind will reduce your tendencies to drift along without a plan.

The importance of goals and objectives

Outcome thinking is a useful term and an effective strategy for becoming organised. What do you want to be doing in five years' time? How about ten years? Do you have a clear plan for your career? Do you have a clear plan for each day? Defining your goals and objectives will help keep you on track and realise your ambitions. They will help you organise your personal and professional life accordingly. Although this book focuses mainly on your medical career it is important to set goals for all areas of your life. Maintaining a healthy work/life balance is a key to success. Devoting yourself to work will impact on your friendships and family life and will not make you a better doctor.

Before you set any objectives, it is important that you understand exactly what purpose they serve.

Measurable objectives increase motivation

So why set objectives? It is always essential to know what you are trying to achieve. Without having an end result in mind you will be unable to create a plan of action which will help you get there. Planning is essential to effective time management. Having planned activities gives shape to your day and allows you to be realistic about what you need to do. It will also develop your motivation and determination as you have identified what is important. Setting goals or objectives may even provide you with a sense of excitement, as the framework of your career becomes evident year by year.

Is there a difference between goals and objectives? Although the terms are often interchanged, there are differences between the two. Goals can be described as being general directions whereas objectives are often conveyed as specific and measurable. This book does not make such distinctions. Do not allow yourself to become distracted or confused by the differences between goals and objectives. Choose the term you prefer and stick with it. In a work context it is more common, perhaps, to talk of objectives, as they often refer to a shorter timeframe, such as one year or less. A goal usually implies a longer timescale and for that reason may be seen as more vague.

An example of a goal might be to become a senior doctor in your chosen field of expertise. An example of an objective might be to complete specific examinations pertinent to your role by the end of the year. Objectives can refer to output, attitudes or behaviour. Most importantly, they can be measured. They are concise and they are specific if set properly. Objectives are used to measure progress and development and are commonly used in the workplace, usually agreed at annual appraisals. You will be given various objectives relating to specific aspects of your role and can cover knowledge, clinical and non-clinical skills. You can also have objectives centred on your personal development. Improving your time management would form the basis of a personal development objective.

Objectives can be thought of as milestones and a means of charting your progress. Without a clear idea of what you are trying to achieve how would you ever know that you had accomplished anything?

As mentioned above, objectives need to be measurable otherwise you cannot accurately identify progress and stay on target to achievement. The following acronym is a useful means of framing your objectives in a way that supports your progress.

SMART stands for specific, measurable, achievable, realistic and time-framed. There are variations on the exact descriptions but the essence is the same.

Time management tip

Make your objectives S.M.A.R.T.

It is important that you make your objectives positive when you create them within the SMART parameters. Do not talk about things that you do not want or that you want to stop. Try and phrase your objectives around things that you do want to achieve.

Ensure they are specific. Be very clear about exactly what you are trying to achieve. Being vague may give you an idea of your general intention but will not provide the motivation you need to achieve them. If your objectives concern examinations, which ones are they specifically? Name them. In case you have not yet realised, the more specific you can be, the clearer you become. Being clear is the key to knowing whether you are going to achieve your outcome.

Your objectives must be measurable so the verbs you use must be clear. A vague objective might describe you 'becoming aware' of time management principles. How will you know you are 'becoming aware'? What would tell you? It will be easier for you to measure your activities if your outcome was better defined. Perhaps being able to identify time management principles would be a far better measure. You would know whether you had achieved your objective because you would either be able to identify the principles or you would not. If you are unsure about whether your objective is measurable, just ask yourself two key questions, "how will I know when I have achieved this objective?" and "what will tell me?"

When setting objectives, make sure you use a practical approach. Are they achievable? In other words are they humanly possible? Would it be achievable for you to walk on the moon in two weeks' time without any training? Of course not, it would not be possible for anyone so the objective is not achievable. The timescale would need to be much longer for you to realise this particular objective.

One of the downfalls for doctors striving for better time management is their inability to be realistic about what they can achieve in the time given. When setting objectives it is important to maintain that realism. Whatever it is you want to achieve in your working or personal life make sure it is realistic for you. It may be possible for someone in the world to achieve it but is it right for you at this particular point in time? You must be realistic about the aims you set yourself or you will become de-motivated.

Having a time-frame can help make an objective realistic and it is always essential to set a deadline. Deadlines are fantastic for focusing one's attention. If you left your objective open ended it could remain a remote possibility, something that would be nice to achieve but in the fullness of time. As you can see, this does not provide sufficient motivation. Deadlines can make objectives loom into view and give you that sense of realisation that you need to get on with things sooner rather than later. So they are a useful mechanism for providing focus, motivation and often the energy that accompanies them. Just be realistic about your deadline and go with your intuition. If the date for completion is at the end of the month you may react with fear which may tell you that there is not enough time. In which case, change the date so that you have a more realistic timescale to work towards.

You may want to have a mix of deadlines. Objectives can be short-term which usually means anywhere from one to three months in their duration. Or they can be mid-term which could be one to three years. Or they could be long term with deadlines for five, ten or twenty years' time. In your working life it will help you to have short and mid-term objectives. Some projects will require your attention now and others can be worked on throughout your year.

Normally you will agree these with your senior but there is nothing to stop you setting your own work objectives if none are forthcoming. As long as they do not undermine your role there is no reason why you should not progress your personal development. Remember to set some objectives or goals for your personal life too, so that you maintain that all important balance. Many doctors have agreed objectives with their senior colleague but they do not conform to the SMART acronym. If this is true for you, ask to meet with your senior again and make your objectives much more specific and ensure that deadlines are agreed by both of you. If you are managing others, ensure you can measure their objectives so that you can, of course, measure performance much more effectively.

When setting SMART objectives do not overwhelm yourself with too many. How many is too many? That will depend upon you of course and what you feel comfortable with. Just be realistic about what you can achieve over the coming months and ensure that your objectives are challenging but accomplishable.

Seeing the bigger picture

Once you have a clear set of objectives to aim for your time management strategies should start to fall into place much more naturally. With your personal targets in mind you can now review what you do. You can identify the activities which move you towards your objectives and make decisions about what to do with the rest. You will feel less inclined to put things off because you realise how important doing them will be to the completion of your objectives. Knowing what you need to achieve will also assist your decision making process. All you need to decide is whether undertaking the particular activity will move you towards or away from your objective. Do not start anything that is likely to lead you away or down a different path other than the one you have planned for yourself. You will become part of a self-fulfilling cycle of success. As you focus and start to see results you will feel a greater sense of achievement which will encourage you to continue. The more you apply good habits and discipline to your work the more results you will see and the cycle continues in a much more positive way than it might be doing now. You have to start somewhere and creating objectives is probably the best place to begin. Give yourself that sense of purpose and then do the tasks that you know will move you closer to achieving your goals or objectives. It doesn't matter what you call them, just have something to aim for! As you begin to see results your stress levels will reduce in a corresponding manner and you will unconsciously become proactive which is a much healthier position for you to be in than reacting all the time to the demands of others.

The importance of action

It is important that you take action and start something, however small. Seize the day and do something positive that will move you forward. Remember that outcomes lead to action and action leads to results. Keep your objectives in your desk drawer or in your wallet. They must be easily accessible because you should look at them every day or at least every week. Constantly remind yourself about what you are being appraised and that will keep you focused. As with all habits this new approach to work and colleagues will get easier over time, however difficult it may seem now. When you have your results in mind it is much easier to get on with those daunting tasks because you are clear about why you are doing them. When you do not know what you are aiming for it is easy to lose sight of what you should be dealing with and you remain a victim of confusion. Take the first steps to clarity today and complete the exercise at the end of this chapter.

Once you have developed your focus strategies and encouraged yourself to take action, you are training yourself to be in the optimum state for time management. The next step will be to manage the expectations of others but again, having objectives will help you do this with ease. You can discuss your objectives with others or at least explain to them why you cannot do them the favour they have just asked of you. Your colleagues will soon learn that you are not being deliberately awkward and they will appreciate your frankness. When they can see that you are genuinely busy with other activities they will approach you less and less. Occasionally you may be able to help them and it would be a good thing to do so but only if it is on your terms and you really do have enough time in your schedule. Hopefully now you can see clearly why having work-related objectives are so powerful in the context of effective time management.

Curb your curiosity if you can. Focus only on the information that you require to meet your objectives. This should help you avoid reading magazines, journals or reports that have little relevance to your role. They may be interesting but they will have to wait. You have much more important things to be getting on with now.

By now you may be feeling more motivated and energised by the thought of becoming focused and clear about what you need to do. However, some of you may still have trouble starting. This is because new habits are not perfectly formed in a matter of hours. They take time to cultivate and they require daily practice. It was mentioned earlier that to take action, however small, is better than taking none.

The ten minute habit

Take heart from the fact that most people are daunted by the prospect of completing a project or task in one attempt. Do not compel yourself to do this. If you spend too much time trying to force your words your mind will probably go blank. The most effective way around this is to utilise the ten minute rule. This means only working on a particular project for a maximum of ten minutes and being able to stop when the time limit is up. When the brain is overloaded it has a tendency to shut down. For example, if you are studying for an exam only the first ten minutes of what you read actually sinks in. It is much the same way with working on a project. Your ideas stop flowing after a while so that is why spending a maximum of ten minutes engaged in a single task is all that you really need to do to be productive. This is a very useful technique for people who have a tendency to put off difficult tasks until the last minute because they are so overwhelmed by the sheer scale of the undertaking.

By limiting yourself to ten minutes your motivation will be much higher and you will be much more likely to begin. When you know that you only have that short amount of time it will feel far less daunting. In order for this to be successful you must make a commitment to ignore incoming e-mails and the ringing telephone. If you are likely to be interrupted by other people walking in and out of your office find a quieter room. When you are ready; check the start time on your watch. Then apply your focus. Concentrate on this one task for the full ten minutes. If this involves writing then do so for the full ten minutes. Do not worry about the content at this stage. It is more important that you are writing and have begun the task than the quality of what you have written. At the end of the ten minute timeframe it is essential that you stop. You must honour the arrangement otherwise you will put yourself off in the future. So walk away and take a short break.

You will be surprised at how much you have written or achieved in the short burst of activity. As it was a limited timeframe, it probably felt less daunting and you will have had enough motivation to start the project. You will have felt that even you can cope with an activity that is only going to last ten minutes. As you were focused you produced a lot more than you ever thought possible.

This rule is a great way of breaking down your resistance to get on with a task. You may even have found that you had more to produce and feel uncomfortable that you have had to stop. What if your brain forgets what you were going to say next? There is no need to worry about this. When you allow your brain to rest by taking a break it is still processing ideas, coming up with answers and improving the words that you have already written as well as shaping the next few paragraphs you are going to write in your next ten minute bout of activity. After your short break you will find that your mind is fresh and you can jump right back in and get ten more minutes of work done. Before you know it you will be well under way with the report or presentation that have been resisting for so long.

Exercise

Using the SMART criteria, create six work related objectives for yourself. Make sure that two of them are short-term, i.e. they have to be complete within the next three months. The remaining four ought to be related to what you would like to achieve within the next twelve months.

Take a piece of paper and write each one down. Ensure they are specific, realistic and easy to measure. Do not forget to add a deadline but make sure the deadline is possible to achieve. Be specific about the date. Do not write, "By the end of next month" but write down the actual date which will make it much more realistic. For example, "By the 31st July" is much more specific and clear.

Keep a copy of your objectives close to hand so that when your bad habits threaten to return you can remind yourself of what you need to achieve over the coming year. Make the commitment to prioritise those activities which help you make progress towards your objective and to delegate or refuse the activities which will not help you achieve that aim.

Summary

- Successful time management is about knowing what you want, basing your decisions on clearly defined objectives and not allowing outside distractions to deter you.

- Developing focus is the foundation for any time management technique.

- Deciding which twenty per cent of your activities yields eighty per cent of your results and doing more of the twenty per cent will focus your mind on what is important.

- Setting measurable objectives will help you foster long-term organisation and provide the motivation for you to be disciplined in what you do each day.

- Before embarking upon any future activity, decide whether it contributes to the achievement of your objectives. If it does not, you should not be doing it.

- Be realistic about the number of objectives you can accomplish.

- Taking small steps towards meeting your objectives is better than no action at all.

- Using the ten minute rule stimulates your brain into focused activity but does not overwhelm it.

Chapter 8   From goals to activities

Aims & objectives

In this chapter you will:

- Learn the benefits of having written goals and objectives
- Break your objectives into smaller sections
- Create 7 sub-categories for your role at work
- Realise the need to record all outstanding tasks in each sub-category
- Break tasks into even smaller activities
- Regain your purpose and motivation by having a full picture of what you need to achieve

The benefits of having written objectives

As the previous chapter stated, a goal or an objective is a desired result, something you want to achieve and which will require specific actions. It is useful in both your personal and working life that you have a mixture of short-term and long-term objectives. In order to develop positive habits of self-organisation you should aim to set objectives for varying time periods: each day, each week, each month and each year. If you set longer term goals, be prepared to review them each year because your circumstances will change and your goals may need some adjustments.

As a doctor you will find it beneficial to write down your goals and objectives. There is a popular urban myth in existence, in various forms, that told of a study conducted at Yale during the 1950s. Supposedly, the students about to graduate were asked if they had goals or ambitions which were written down. Only three percent confirmed they had committed their ambitions to paper. Apparently, ten years later when the researchers followed up their project, the three percent were earning nearly ten times as much as the individuals who had not written down their goals. Those individuals who had formulated goals in their mind were still earning a great deal more than the graduates who had left without forming any goals for themselves at all.

No proof can be found to substantiate this story, but whether this is myth or fact, it is still worth considering the benefits of having written goals or objectives. The very act of writing them down helps to internalise them and make them memorable. The practical advantages are obvious. Being able to refer to a list of work-related objectives for the coming year is invaluable. Such a list will help any doctor stay on track and in line with his or her purpose. When you are able to remind yourself each week of what you have committed to achieve, then you are far less likely to be distracted by other projects or favours. You can retain your motivation and determination to achieve.

Breaking objectives into smaller steps

However, it may be difficult for you to maintain your motivation when the objective you have set yourself or that has been set for you may seem too large an undertaking. You may feel daunted by the sheer size of the objective and these feelings will be doubled if the objective carries a high level of complexity. For some of you, your objectives will extend over a longer period of time and stretch out over a two or three year period. These objectives are also difficult to commence because where do you start? It will be challenging to remain focused when you do not even know where to begin. Therefore, it makes perfect sense for you to break down your objectives into smaller, more manageable chunks.

One useful way of doing this is to divide your life into categories. These categories should encompass your personal life as well as your working life in order to give you a complete picture of the obligations you need to meet but most of them must relate to your professional life. The categories are designed to help you reach your objectives as you will find it easier to continue the positive habit of setting priorities and give you a continual overview of where you should be focusing your attention and effort. The categories you decide upon will contain all the related tasks to a particular objective or set of objectives. This will help you focus on your workload in a more organised manner and afford you complete control over your working and personal life.

Do not over-categorise

The categories you choose constitute the main areas of your life and will help you put your activities into better perspective. Ideally you should have a maximum of nine categories, two of which will be focused on your personal life and the remainder on your working life. If you have more than nine, you will limit your ability to keep track of progress. The optimum number is seven but you will find the number that is right for you. These categories will be headings for related tasks and activities, all designed to help you reach your specific objectives or goals. Make sure that your category headings are quite broad and able to combine related key areas of your life, such as "family and friends".

People have different ways of establishing the category headings that are right for them. Some people review all the things they have to do and group together related tasks. Then they choose the most appropriate title for that particular category. Or they think about what they do in general, on a daily and weekly basis and try and group related tasks together, before giving each group a category name.

Other people begin by reviewing their objectives. They look at the overall requirements of their work role and also what they want to achieve. From there they are able to identify the key areas of work within which they need to concentrate their efforts. It does not matter which approach you take as long as you are able to identify up to nine key headings into which you can group your tasks.

Why do it this way?

Remember you are now cultivating new habits of working and trying to establish strategies which enable you to manage your time in the most effective way. Creating sub-categories for your work role, in particular, will help you maintain the practice of setting priorities and focusing your energy where it is needed the most.

No two doctors will have the same categories. It will very much depend upon your specialty and the stage at which you find yourself in your career. Having said that, it is probable that all doctors will find it beneficial to have a category for clinical duties, and one for personal and professional development. If you are a senior doctor you will have responsibilities towards junior members of staff. It will be your responsibility to ensure that your team is effective and motivated so that they can deliver the best possible service for patients. Therefore, one of your key categories should be allocated to 'staff' or 'people'.

Most doctors will need a category entitled 'administration' as this will group together any paperwork activities and work rotas. It will also cover sickness rotas and holiday arrangements. The maintenance of patient notes is likely to be part of this category. Any outstanding activities relating to patient records can be annotated here for eventual scheduling in to the diary.

What other categories can you think of which relate specifically to your role? Are you responsible for or involved with a particular complex or large project? Perhaps you are working on more than one project? Perhaps you are part of a project team or leading it. Whatever your circumstance you will need a category relating to 'Projects' so that you can co-ordinate any outstanding related tasks here. To make it even easier for you to manage, you may decide to have category headings for each project, if they are particularly large. Senior doctors will also be responsible for improvements to their service. This will undoubtedly be a category in its own right as there will be many activities associated with this ongoing responsibility.

Other categories could include Clinical Audit or Research. Again, these may also be regarded as one-off projects. It will be up to you to decide how you wish to organise your commitments.

It is worth noting at this stage that category headings will change from time to time and you may decide upon one approach but realise, after some time that it is not working for you. If this happens try an alternative way. For example, you may initially decide that it is easier to group all your project tasks into one heading of 'Projects', but over time you realise that you cannot successfully manage your activities in this way. You may then decide to have a category heading per project and organise yourself that way. As new responsibilities occur in your role you will find that you need to add or change existing category headings.

If you are involved with financial matters you will probably need a category devoted to 'Finance'. This is where any budget tasks would be allocated or business case information. Again, use your judgement to decide the most appropriate headings and you may well base this initially, on your existing tasks.

If you attend a number of meetings or regularly work with other teams you may want a category that covers internal communication or working relationships. As stated earlier, Personal Development should definitely be a category heading for you and this would include any personal objectives or goals you have set yourself. Of course this could include any activities associated with your professional development too. Training courses which attract CPD points could form objectives which can be included in this category or you may want a specific category for Professional Development, relating to any activities which form part of your career progression.

Perhaps you have been delegated a particular area of responsibility? You may decide that it warrants its own category. For example, if you had been asked to represent colleagues or sit on specific steering committees, you may decide that it would be easier for you to focus on these tasks if they were contained in a category heading of their own. Perhaps you are keen on teaching and would like to develop this part of your role more fully? Teaching could definitely be a category within which you set yourself some clear objectives.

As you can see there are a number of ways to categorise your life and only you can decide what is meaningful to you but the examples given above should help you get started.

Remember to set aside at least two categories for non-work activities, such as 'Friends and Family' or 'Health and Fitness'. Once you have created a maximum of nine categories it is a good idea to share your thoughts with your senior colleague, the person to whom you report. They may hold a different perspective and want you to focus on other areas of your role. It is better to establish this early on before you begin the process of organising yourself and your time effectively and you may gain insights into where you have been going wrong previously.

Record all outstanding tasks in each category

Now you should have clarity about the key areas of your work and personal life that require your attention. If you have applied the 80/20 rule as well, you may have been able to create categories for your high yielding activities or at least have grouped them together into one category. For the more visual among you, you may want to adopt a similar process to your priority setting method and use a mind map for each category heading. Place the category heading in the middle of the page and now write down all the tasks associated with it on the rest of the page.

Writing down the tasks which have to be completed in each category is the next part of the process in breaking your work into smaller pieces, enabling you to avoid the anxiety of facing a huge commitment in one go. This should be a relatively easy process. Remember that you are not setting priorities at this stage. You are merely organising your commitments into a manageable framework and ensuring that your activities are focused on achieving your objectives. If you can develop the habit of doing this regularly, you will then naturally start to set priorities from within each category, asking yourself if the particular task is essential and requires your immediate attention. Most of them will not and will sit neatly in the 'essential but not immediate' mind map. This level of organisation enables you to work effectively with tasks from each category and you should be able to schedule some into each working week.

Be clear about your tasks. They need to be as specific as your objectives and will benefit from having a deadline. Never be vague when it comes to time management or you will always underestimate your workload and how long it takes. When you write down the task on your category mind map, write down a complete sentence and include a completion date. Doing so will help you set priorities each week.

Examples of tasks which may occur in the administration category could be agreeing the next shift rota, completing patient notes, filing old paperwork, dealing with patient complaints and so on.

Attending a time management training course is a task that could be included in your Personal Development or Professional Development category.

As your tasks are scheduled and completed they can be removed from your mind map. Some tasks will be ongoing and occur each week, in which case, just ensure you schedule them as a regular activity in your weekly diary and leave them on the category mind map so that you remember to schedule them each week or however frequently they occur.

Break your tasks into smaller actions for clarity

Now that you have up to nine categories of focus, with objectives and tasks relating to each one, you are in a very strong position in terms of your personal effectiveness. However, if necessary, it is possible to break your tasks down even further and for many doctors who are unable to manage their time well, this is a very helpful final step. Poor time managers often under estimate how long a task will take and this is because they have not considered the activities associated with the task. A good example is the task of giving an appraisal to a member of staff. At first glance this would appear to be one task and someone may mistakenly schedule it in the diary and allocate one hour to it. In reality, there are a number of activities associated with giving an appraisal. The necessary paperwork for the individual has to be collated, the previous year's objectives must be obtained and feedback from colleagues must be sought regarding the individual's performance throughout the year. Sometimes a pre-meeting has to be arranged with the individual in order to explain the process to them and outline what is expected of them at the appraisal meeting. A room must be booked, if appropriate, or a quiet place found so that the confidential discussion can take place without interruption. All paperwork must be read and a new set of objectives thought about in advance. There is much to be done before finally, the appraisal meeting itself can take place. Nor do associated activities end with the meeting. There will be additional activities after the appraisal has been held and all of them must be noted or they may be overlooked and not scheduled. It is easy to see that taking the further step of breaking tasks down into component activities is a necessary part of the process and essential to effective time management and personal organisation.

How do you record the activities and where do you keep them? Again it is a matter of personal choice but this book recommends keeping a 'to do' list of activities which are related to one another and to one specific task. For every task on the category mind map there should be an accompanying list of activities and these can be clipped behind the mind map for future reference. Rather than leaving everything to the last minute, you will now be in a position each week to review what is outstanding on your activity lists and schedule each small action as you wish into your diary.

Seeing the full commitment

This method yields a number of benefits to you. Not only do you gain a true picture of your commitments and workload, but you have also broken them down into manageable actions. Some of the actions given in the appraisal example might only take a few minutes and can easily be scheduled into a busy day. The same will be true of your activities. This allows you to get ahead and progress even the longer-term of your commitments. There is no excuse not to get on with your tasks and you will gain a real sense of achievement as, little by little, you start to reduce your workload. When the actions are many but small you will not feel so overwhelmed by them and, therefore, should feel motivated enough to progress them. You will be surprised at the number of small actions you can fit into each working week. Tick off each action as you do it as that will also help you realise just how much you are achieving.

You may decide that some of your actions can be delegated, saving you even more time for your high-yielding activities, but remember to schedule time in your week in order to delegate properly. Some actions will be so simple that not much explanation will be necessary. Others, however, may require a more formal or structured briefing so even the act of delegating must be considered a task and broken down into smaller actions. Again, a time and a place must be arranged for the briefing and follow up meetings must be considered. When you approach all your activities in this way, you will soon get used to this method of working and will enjoy the efficiencies it brings you.

Develop a weekly process

To maintain your ongoing personal organisation you will review your situation each week and update or amend your tasks and activities as appropriate. You will set your priorities for the week and schedule in activities accordingly. If you continue to be realistic about how long each action will take and build in some contingency, just in case, you will regain so much peace of mind and control of your life. Always leave gaps in each day so that you can handle unexpected events and the inevitable interruptions.

Understand that you may find this new way of working a challenge at first. It takes one month to foster a new habit but this one is definitely worth it. The benefits far outweigh any burden associated with the effort of becoming organised and of course, you can build in this activity into your weekly schedule, just like any other task. You may want to have an early start each Monday for the first month so that you can start to practise your new habit in relative peace before your shift begins. If you commute, you have a perfect opportunity for using some transition time to organise yourself without interruption.

You will soon find your preferred method and do not worry if you do not follow all the advice given to you in this book. As long as you are more effective and more organised you will reap the benefits and so will your colleagues who will be impacted in a much more positive way than previously.

Exercise

Create the appropriate categories for your working life and include two categories that relate to your personal life. You can either refer to your existing objectives and shape your categories from them or group some objectives into one major area. If you do not have any formal objectives you can still think about which accomplishments you would like to achieve over the coming months and year.

The other way of deciding on key areas of your role would be to review your outstanding tasks and group them together into general headings. If you find yourself with more than nine, see if you can amalgamate some headings together, otherwise you will overwhelm yourself. It should be possible for you to have nine or less if you have successfully dealt with your crises, as advised in the early part of this book. You must deal with the existing problems before trying to organise yourself as part of your ongoing self-management.

Now list all your tasks associated with each category. Use the mind map system if you wish. Ensure your tasks are specific, time-framed and written as a complete sentence. If you prefer lists, make sure that your task list is attached to the category sheet to which it pertains.

Some of your tasks will require a further break down into specific and smaller activities. On a separate sheet of paper, write down the task and underline it. List all the actions that you need to complete in order to achieve the task. Do this with all your tasks.

This exercise will take you some time but it will be worth it in order for you to gain true clarity about what your workload involves. This exercise should be repeated each week but will be much quicker to do as you will be only updating or deleting items from your existing lists.

When you are ready, review all your actions in the context of the priority setting method and start to schedule a few into your diary for the coming week.

Stay focused, stay determined and feel excited about how organised you are becoming. Cross off each action as you complete it, or at the end of each working day and savour that sense of satisfaction. You have earned it.

Summary

- Writing down your objectives helps to internalise them and bring them into focus.

- Objectives can be daunting due to their complexity, size or deadline.

- Organising your life into nine main categories helps you focus your activities.

- To achieve a work-life balance you should include two categories relating to your personal life.

- Setting objectives or goals in all categories of your life gives you a sense of purpose and balance.

- Breaking objectives into smaller chunks makes them more manageable and, therefore, more motivating.

- Working out the tasks associated with each objective and category gives a true sense of what needs to be done, by whom and by when.

- Breaking tasks down into actions allows you to be realistic about what needs to be done.

- It is important to list all actions and attach the list to the task sheet in order to track ongoing progress.

- Breaking down tasks into smaller actions allows many more to be scheduled into the diary each week and far quicker progress can be made on all objectives or projects, no matter how daunting.

- The effective management of organising one's workload into achievable actions enhances the ability to control stress levels and significantly reduce anxiety.

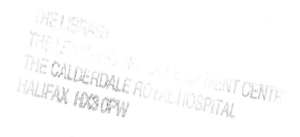

Chapter 9 Learn to delegate

Aims & objectives

In this chapter you will:

- Be able to define the act of delegation
- Understand the reason for delegating
- Explore your own resistance to it.
- Identify the many benefits of delegating
- Learn how to overcome your resistance
- Work out what can and what cannot be delegated
- Understand the process of delegating effectively

If you have been following the advice in this book and attempting to implement some of the techniques, you will have already begun to re-organise your workload according to priorities and break down larger projects into more manageable sizes. It is essential to sort out the current chaos but what will be far more important for you now is to prevent the situation from happening again. If you have been reading this book in chronological order you will see that it transitions from dealing with the current situation to thinking about long-term strategies for self organisation.

Being able to delegate some of your work is obviously one of the best ways to claw back your precious time. Using the prioritisation tools outlined in the previous chapters you now know that there is a whole category of jobs or tasks that can be given away. All the tasks that are not essential to you but appear to be important or urgent to other people can be delegated. Any activity which has that sense of 'now' about it and yet will have little impact on your aims and objectives can be carried out by someone other than you without any feelings of guilt. Successful time managers recognise the entire category of 'not essential but immediate' items as a gift because all of the activities within this group can be performed by someone else and immediately free up time to do items which take a higher priority. It makes perfect sense to delegate. Yet so many doctors struggle with this concept.

Many doctors find themselves wholly unable to hand over work to anyone else, despite the fact that the obvious rewards of much needed time would become available. What makes it so difficult for doctors to entrust responsibilities and tasks to other people? What is stopping you?

Defining delegation

Perhaps it would be best to start with an explanation of delegation and understand what it really means. A common definition states that delegation means assigning a certain task to another person providing proper authorisation. Whilst definitions tend to focus on managers delegating to junior members of the team, this does not have to be the case. Peers can delegate to peers but probably phrase the request in a different way. True delegation needs to be effective and effective delegation encourages ownership of responsibility on the part of the person to whom you are delegating.

Successful delegation in simple words means using the power and willingness of other people to work hard and help you get things done. Other people could be subordinates, colleagues within the department or teammates. If you can enlist the assistance of another individual in accomplishing a task, you can complete large volumes of work in less time. As you can see the art of delegation is a hugely significant skill underpinning effective time management.

There are valid reasons for learning how to delegate. Not only does it regain precious time for you which can be spent on higher priorities and move you towards your objectives, but it is a key skill, central to both time management and leadership. No matter what stage of your medical career you find yourself, learning how to delegate to others is an invaluable tool which will serve you well the more senior you become.

The barriers to delegating

Many doctors resist delegating so it is worth exploring the many barriers that are cited when discussing this skill.

The most common reason given for not delegating is a lack of trust on the part of the delegator. They are usually hindered by the thought that the other person will not perform the delegated job well or properly and that they, the delegator, will have to spend even more time in the end, rectifying the mistakes of the other person. Some doctors believe that it takes too long to explain the delegated task. They think that they could have done the job in the time it takes to explain to another person what has to be done. Some doctors feel guilty for imposing more work on their colleagues or junior members of staff. They fear they will become unpopular or might gain a reputation among the team for giving away too much of their work. In fact some doctors believe that might be true and question how much of their role they will have left if they delegate their tasks to the team. Some senior doctors have expressed, anecdotally, their concerns of delegating a task to someone who performs it better than they can. They are worried at being exposed in this way. As you can see there are many barriers to delegating and nearly all of them self-imposed. What are your reasons? Can you relate to the ones given in this chapter? Even if some of them are potentially true, you must find ways of overcoming them or you will slip back into old habits and take on too much and worse still, take on the work of other people which really doesn't concern you or help you achieve your objectives. Some people manage to delegate perfectly well. If they can, so can you.

For junior doctors the most common reason cited is that of not having anyone to whom they can delegate. If that is your reason try thinking of it in a different way. Move away from your current interpretation of the word delegating which you probably associate with giving work to someone more junior than you. Consider the true definition of delegation which is enlisting the help and support of another person. That person does not have to be your junior. They could well be your colleague or peer or someone from the larger team who is not a doctor. There are many non-clinical tasks which can be delegated.

Limiting beliefs and assumptions

It is clear to see from the resistance to delegating outlined above that most reasons for not sharing tasks with other people are based on individual assumptions about how the process may be perceived and around how the delegator may be perceived too. There are also anxieties around how the recipient may perform the delegated task. However, perception is not actual truth. It is merely individual reality, based on personal beliefs. The processes of perception routinely alter what humans see. When people view something with a preconceived idea about it, their behaviour will be greatly influenced.

A person's knowledge, experience and beliefs create his or her reality as much as the truth, because the human mind can only contemplate that to which it has been exposed. It is easy to understand then, how doctors will be reluctant to delegate if they hold the beliefs and assumptions outlined above. If you think another person cannot be trusted to do the task properly then the chances of you delegating that specific job to that particular person is remote. If you believe that you will not be liked by someone because you have delegated a job to them that thought will also prevent you from taking that necessary action. Perhaps it is worth examining your reluctance to delegate. Are your reasons based on fact or do you hold some limiting beliefs around the skill? Do you harbour unfounded assumptions about other people? Remember the old saying that 'assumption makes an ass out of you and me'. Do not assume that junior colleagues cannot cope with a new duty. Do not assume that they will resist a new responsibility when it is offered to them. Do not assume that your colleagues will stop respecting you if you ask for their help and support. Understand that most of the barriers to delegating are psychological and unfounded. Work out what yours are and think about developing a strategy for overcoming your negative association. You may prefer to think about the consequences to you if you continue not to delegate some of your work. How will your situation improve if you continue to accept work that holds no significance for you or cannot share a small section of your work with others?

Take a moment to write down all your objections to delegating. Leave space beneath each one so that you can return to them at a future point with a solution.

The benefits of delegating

Sometimes talking about the gains of utilising a skill can help overcome perceived barriers. Examining the benefits of delegating may be a useful way of understanding why you need to master this skill. If you change your perceptions of delegating in the positive light of the advantages it offers you will be much more likely to try. Probably the most important reason for delegating is to develop the skills of other people as well as yourself. As a senior doctor you have a responsibility to develop everyone in the team, particularly your juniors, and you will be able to delegate both clinical and non-clinical skills. All juniors deserve the opportunity to develop their skills, so it becomes a pre-requisite for you to delegate some tasks to them. A great source of dissatisfaction among team members is when they are not given enough to do. It does not take long for them to suspect you do not trust them and this can quickly create a negative atmosphere and a mistrust of you in return. Senior doctors hold a position of leadership and will be expected to delegate to all the team. If you are senior, you must uphold the team's purpose and ensure that all objectives are achieved. You must understand that most of the individuals in your team want a challenge and will be highly motivated by undertaking tasks and projects that are unfamiliar to them but stretch them beyond their perceived capabilities.

If you are not yet leading a team you will still have many opportunities to delegate and you can also regard this process as a way of developing colleagues. Or you can perceive delegating as a way of sharing knowledge and skills with your peers.

Do not lose sight of why you need to delegate. A very obvious benefit is the amount of time it will earn you back. This is time you could be better spending on the tasks and actions that are more important for you and for the accomplishment of your objectives. If ever you feel a resistance to delegation rise up within you, remember how much time you will claim back and let this spur you on. The whole point is to use the time available in the most effective manner and this inevitably means encouraging other people to take on some responsibilities that you do not have time for. You need to work smarter, not harder, so if you can master the skill of delegating, you will be able to organise your time more effectively.

Each individual in the team will have their strengths and weaknesses. If you have a role which encompasses some form of leadership, then you need to take an overview of what the team, as a whole, needs to achieve. What kind of service do you want to provide and is everyone being utilised in the best possible way? If not, delegation can be used to play to the strengths of the team. There may be someone who really enjoys the tasks you dislike and would appreciate the opportunity of undertaking them. There may be individuals who are better suited to a particular type of work than you. Do not be threatened by this. See it as the opportunity it really is and use it wisely. Do not let your ego get in the way of effective time management. If someone else can do the task better than you, for whatever reason, then it makes sense to let them take that action. Remember you need to reclaim as much time back as you can, so do not hesitate to give tasks to a willing participant.

As mentioned earlier, delegating is a great way to demonstrate trust in others, no matter whether you are senior or still in training. It is a useful way of building trust at the same time. Individuals trust your judgement in them and are flattered by it and they also begin to trust their capabilities as they take on more and more new tasks or responsibilities. The benefits to the whole team are obvious when skills, knowledge and responsibility are spread among the individuals. Motivation increases with empowerment and the team responsible for delivering a patient focused service should be able to do so with ease. Delegation is about ownership and if it is done effectively, each individual will accept ownership for the action and in doing so, develop their skills on a professional level.

It is important to acknowledge another benefit of delegating. You will primarily be giving away work that you should not be doing in the first place. This is work you have agreed to take on before you had clear sight of what you were meant to be focusing on. Delegating allows you the opportunity to get that work done, but not at the expense of your own time. Whilst you do not want to pass on the obligation to someone else, it is a necessary evil to free up your own precious time and should serve as a deterrent to giving in to future requests.

Think of the benefit of being able to progress so much more work than if you continued to do everything yourself. A lot more can be achieved through delegating and you will stand a much greater chance of fulfilling your objectives. That has got to be your number one priority as you will be appraised on this at some point during the year.

There are solutions to every problem so it is worth now returning to the barriers discussed earlier and finding answers to help overcome them. As they are personal and limiting beliefs, unique to each person, this book can only offer suggestions for change. Feel free to get creative and think your way out of your reluctance.

Overcoming common barriers

I cannot trust anyone to do the job properly

Effective delegation means taking the time to explain the job or task fully to the person who is expected to carry it out on your behalf. A rushed conversation while on the way to another commitment is not acceptable. Proper time must be allocated and a thorough briefing given. This will involve stating the desired outcome and may also include explaining the process step by step. The process of delegating is not complete until the recipient of the information feels confident and able to undertake the work alone.

I will spend more time rectifying the mistakes of others

See the advice given above. Similar rules apply. If you delegate properly you are less likely to have to rectify mistakes at the end of the process. If you do not give all the information required to do the job then it is very likely that the work will not be done properly and you will have to sort out the confusion. Poor delegation leads to poor results.

It takes too long to explain – it is quicker to do it myself

Do you really believe that to be true? It takes a curious logic to decide that doing every job oneself is quicker than giving some work to other people! Making time initially will save time in the longer term. The person to whom you delegate may require quite a bit of your time while they learn how to do the task you require, but after that they should be able to do the particular job without your continued assistance. If the task is a one off then make sure you delegate to someone with strong enough capability, someone who will not take too long to brief and, therefore, not take up too much of your time. As you now know, however, there are many low risk activities which can be delegated without time consuming effort. In all cases, be clear about what you want and, if appropriate, how the task should be performed. If the 'how' does not matter, let the individual approach the task in their own way. Always give a deadline. When you have delegated clearly and the recipient indicates their understanding, walk away and focus on your priorities.

Delegating makes me feel guilty

There is no need to feel guilty about delegating work if you are doing so for the right reasons. Your colleagues or juniors may be busy but so are you. Do not let their workload prevent you from seeking their support. Other people will always tell you how busy they are but perhaps this is due to a lack of effective time management on their part. When developing a junior member of the team, you may well be called upon to prioritise their workload for them. If you need to give someone extra work you may have to review their schedule with them and agree new priorities. Feeling guilty about delegating is a waste of time and energy. Instead, try focusing on what needs to be done by you and then work out what could usefully and helpfully be done by others. If you explain your reasons carefully to the person whose support you seek they are much more likely to understand and be willing to help. If you do not communicate effectively then you may cause some resentment, due to misunderstanding.

People won't like me

This is another limiting belief and quite unfounded. People do not stop liking another individual just because they have been asked to do some work for them. How many colleagues do you know who are disliked because they have delegated some work? The team may often moan or gossip but that is human nature and it does not mean dislike or resentment. As stated in the previous paragraph, if you delegate with honourable intentions, people will not think the worse of you. If you use delegating as a way of ridding yourself of all the jobs you dislike or as a means of having very little to do yourself as a result, then you deserve the disrespect of your colleagues. However, if you delegate because you need to focus on your priorities and you can help someone else develop a new skill at the same time, then you are using the skill wisely. Not all delegated tasks will help others develop but they still have to be done and in this situation a proper briefing is necessary so that the perception, by others, of you avoiding your work can be prevented.

I won't have a job to do if I delegate

This is another limiting belief which is wholly unfounded. You need to delegate because you have too much work to do already. Some jobs you delegate will help other people develop their skills. Other, more minor, tasks or activities will simply allow others to offer their support and allow you to get on with the commitments which are most important to you. In either scenario you will still have a large part of your job to do.

What if the other person is better than me?

Do not be distracted by your ego. It shouldn't really matter who does the job the best, only that the work is being done. Keep focused on the outcome, not the person performing the task. Play to the strengths of others who will probably enjoy the delegated duties and enable you to utilise your areas of strength on other activities.

I don't have anyone to delegate to

For junior doctors this is the most common reason cited for not delegating. If that is your reason try thinking of it in a different way. Move away from your current interpretation of the word delegating which you probably associate with giving work to someone more junior than you.

Consider the true definition of delegation which is enlisting the help and support of another person. That person does not have to be your junior. They could well be your colleague or peer or someone from the larger team who is not a doctor. There are many non-clinical tasks which can be delegated.

How to delegate – The process:
Setting outcomes

It is important that you are clear in your mind about what you want done. You need to think about this beforehand in order for you to be clear in your communication. Delegate major tasks as well as minor ones but be clear that major tasks and projects will require more of your time and the delegation method requires more information and detail from you. Make the delegation meeting one of your 'essential but not immediate' items and assign it the appropriate amount of time in your weekly schedule.

The briefing meeting

Do not delegate in a rushed or haphazard manner. Your colleagues must be prepared for the work you want them to do. At the briefing meeting, once you have discussed your desired outcome you must agree together about the resources needed to carry out the work. Resources may include finance, equipment, training and the co-operation of other departments. Make sure that the person concerned has everything they need to carry out the task. This includes authority. Make other people, including those outside the team, aware that you have delegated authority to your colleague if it is required for them to do the assigned work. There is nothing more frustrating for someone than not being able to get things done because they do not hold formal authority. Make it easy for them and remove the barrier. Delegate everything necessary.

Monitoring

As stated before, effective delegation is not about giving someone a job to do and then walking away, abdicating all accountability. Proper delegation must include processes for monitoring progress. You must be aware of developments at all stages of the work if it is of a complex or long term nature. How much you monitor will also depend upon the capability and experience of the person you delegate to. If you are delegating to junior members of the team then you will need to review their progress on a regular basis. If, however, you are sharing work with a colleague, this will not be necessary. However, you should still agree with your colleague that some sort of monitoring or update process will be useful in order for you to retain awareness. For short or easy tasks and activities you will probably decide that only an end review is required when you can be updated regarding the final outcome.

Reviewing

At the end of any project or major delegated activity it is useful to hold a formal review. Similar to the briefing process it is ideal to hold a meeting where the two of you can properly reflect on events and discuss any points for improvement. If the person to whom you delegated is a junior member of your team then you will probably adopt a coaching and supportive style of managing, allowing the individual to tell you what happened, what they would do differently in the future and how they felt about the project. When complex delegated tasks are successful, it is very motivating and empowering for the person. If things do not go quite as anticipated, it is important to make time to talk things through and offer your support. Do not consider this a waste of your time. It is an important way of developing team skills and ultimately will lead to improved job performance.

Evaluating the results

This is a time of reflection on your part. Consider whether your method of delegating was successful. Did you delegate to the right person given the timeframe? Did you delegate with enough notice or did you make it difficult for the person to prepare? Was the amount of support you gave sufficient or did you remain too attached to the project? By making the time to evaluate the success of the delegated tasks you will save time in future by improving your delegation techniques.

Praising and encouraging

Although this may seem obvious, many doctors report that they do not receive much, if any, praise and yet it is a great motivator when given sincerely. When you are developing someone's skills by delegating unfamiliar tasks to them, demonstrating your support is critical. Giving praise and being prepared to listen to concerns and give advice are all powerful ways of building confidence. Confidence is key to all performance issues and once you have instilled it in your colleagues you will be able to delegate to them on a regular basis. If you are asking a colleague to help you with work it will be important to acknowledge their support and assistance and thank them accordingly.

What cannot be delegated?

It is unfair to delegate only the jobs you do not like or which are unpleasant. You must delegate any task which is not your priority and that may well include the simple jobs you enjoy. When you delegate it is important during your briefing meeting that you make it clear that the responsibility and authority for completing the task is delegated also. However, what you should not delegate is accountability for the task. Accountability is a similar term to responsibility, so how may accountability be accurately defined?

U.S. President Harry S. Truman made famous a slogan which he had on his desk bearing the words, 'The buck stops here.' The meaning of this statement indicated that responsibility was not passed on beyond that point. It meant that Truman never 'passed the buck' to anyone else but always held ultimate responsibility for the way the country was governed.

In delegation terms, accountability is the acknowledgement of responsibility even when the actions may be of other people. If you delegate a task, it is still you who must answer to someone senior and report on progress. Although many doctors feel this justifies the pointlessness of delegating, all it really means is that you must ensure you are kept fully informed of progress, problems and the ultimate outcome of the task. Do not delegate and walk away, never again to enquire about how the task is progressing. You must review the situation regularly and be able to update senior staff with facts. You must also be prepared to deal with the consequences of problems which may arise. If deadlines are missed it is you who must provide explanations, so delegate properly and be clear about what you expect from your colleagues in return.

Exercise

Go through the outstanding tasks which you have prioritised into the 'not essential but immediate' category or mind map.

Taking each one in turn, decide to whom you could best delegate the action.

For more complex tasks, assess the capabilities and willingness of the person to whom you wish to delegate. What information might they need from you before proceeding? How much support will they need, if any?

Now review some earlier exercises where you created action lists for each task associated with your objectives. Decide which of the small and non-time consuming actions can be done by other people quickly and without impacting upon their workload significantly.

Spread the delegated tasks to more than one colleague or team member so as to maintain the balance of workload among the team.

Prepare a complete list of actions, assignees and the deadlines and ensure that you have delegated as much as you possibly can.

Summary

- Delegation means using the power and willingness of other people to help you get things done.
- Delegating gives you back the time you need to focus on your important priorities.
- It provides a great opportunity for other members of the team to develop their professional skills.
- Most barriers to delegating are self-imposed and based on assumptions about negative perceptions by others.
- Identifying the benefits of delegating can overcome that resistance.

- Any tasks in 'not essential but immediate' can be delegated

- It is important to implement the proper process for delegating tasks, which involves a briefing meeting and an agreement about resources. You should also be prepared to review progress and evaluate the results. Never abdicate your accountability for the delegated work.

Chapter 10   Prevention is better than cure – learn to say no

Aims & objectives

In this chapter you will:

- Explore the popular misconceptions about saying no

- Understand what makes it so difficult

- Identify the 3 key influencing skills and decide which is your preference

- Understand how an assertive approach will help you say no in future

- Learn how to negotiate your way to a refusal

- Be able to challenge requests

- Overcome your anxiety about what others may think of you

If you feel guilty about delegating to other people, the answer lies in not placing yourself in that position in the first place. If you have no one to whom you can delegate the same advice applies. The alternative is to stop accepting other people's work or carrying out favours for colleagues. Saying no will be a useful weapon in the quest for more effective time management. Even if you prioritise your workload as shown earlier, your efforts will be wasted if you continue to do other people's work. How many times have you said yes to things you wanted to say no to? Was it easier to give in? Would saying no have made you feel guilty or worried that you would upset someone? Did you imagine that if you said no you would have burdened someone else with the delegated task and that would be unfair? Consequently you ended up doing some work that was not essential for you and did not help you achieve your priorities. Conversely, it prevented you from meeting your priorities and objectives. Having made such an effort at becoming organised, it is important to adopt two key skills and behaviours which prevent the previous situation from happening again. One new skill is delegation and the other is assertiveness.

Popular misconceptions about saying no

In medicine there is a strong feeling among junior doctors that they cannot say no to senior colleagues. As with any junior role many individuals feel unable to refuse any request from their boss, who in this context could be any senior ranking doctor.

Senior doctors, also, may find it hard to say no to colleagues because they believe it would be rude to refuse such requests. Many people believe that their refusal will be held against them and they will be viewed as lazy or unsupportive by their peers. Rather than run the risk of becoming unpopular, doctors continue to say yes to tasks that are irrelevant and unhelpful to them.

However, by continually giving in to others and taking on more work than you can realistically cope with, you are wasting time. Making commitments to others means neglecting your own commitments. Very often the result is anxiety, frustration and resentment. You may find yourself trapped by the non-essential activities that others have asked you to do. You can see your own work increasing but are unable to deal with it within the timeframe you desire. Worst of all is that instead of being respected and valued by your colleagues or seniors, you will be taken for granted and viewed as an easy target for the delegation of unwanted tasks.

You may believe that it is impolite to say no and you may want to be popular with your team, viewed as a reliable and helpful resource. But this approach does not help you manage your time appropriately. It does not earn you the respect you hope for. In fact it may earn you the reputation of a poor time manager, one who cannot manage priorities effectively and is always staying late to catch up. Your stress levels will rise and each day you will become less effective.

Saying no will save you time. You will have very few items in the 'not essential but immediate' category and this will leave you free to work on the essential pieces of work, the ones which are a higher priority for you. This book does not advocate you saying no for the sake of it. If you have planned your week properly and you genuinely do have spare time then it is preferable to be able to help out a colleague. However, saying no will allow you to focus on the things that matter most to you. It will also reduce your levels of stress that a burgeoning workload can bring. To be a safe doctor for your patients you need to be a healthy doctor and one who is in control of a manageable daily workload.

Why saying no can be difficult

If you think back to your childhood you may find it harder to recall incidences of you being afraid to say no. Children do not usually have such a problem! If they do not want to do something they make it perfectly clear. They do not worry about what their parents or teachers will think of them. It does not even occur to them to think in this way. What they focus on is ensuring that they do not do whatever it is they are resisting. Some children can be so forceful that they win the power struggle and it is their less assertive parents who back away from the argument.

However, as we grow up we are taught that it is wrong to say no. We are conditioned to believe that we must do as we are told or face the consequences. It is clear to see then that saying no is a learned behaviour and for many people becomes an unconscious, ingrained habit.

In some cultures it is considered rude to say no in which case another way must be found. In these circumstances it may be more effective for a discussion to take place about the order of priorities, or for an explanation to be offered about the amount of work you are already committed to. If you find yourself working in a country that is not your native home and it is one where it is acceptable to refuse requests, then it is advisable that you try and learn to be more assertive or you will be at the continual mercy of stronger and more forceful personalities. Until you learn to say no to other people in favour of your own commitments you will be over burdened with work and likely to be suffering from stress and anxiety. If you do not address the situation you may present a real risk to your patients.

Understanding influencing styles

The term 'influencing styles' relates to communication and refers to how strongly messages can be conveyed to other people. Traditionally, influence is described as the ability of one person to get others to behave in a particular way or to carry out certain actions. This would be easy to understand in the context of delegating and asking for the support of colleagues. However, it is equally relevant to discuss influencing skills in the context of refusing requests because we are actually talking about the strength of the communication.

There are 3 levels or strengths of influencing skills. The first is known as passivity or passiveness and is the weakest of the influencing skills.

What does it mean to be passive?

Being passive means not standing up for yourself or your rights. It means not being able to express your needs and feelings to other people and this inability often leads to frustration and anger. Passive people usually put other people first and they focus on pleasing other people. They believe that other people's needs are more important than their own. The ultimate aim of passive behaviour and approaches is to avoid conflict. It is easy to see why a passive person is less able to say no to the requests of others and can be overburdened with work, resulting in poor time management.

What does it mean to be aggressive?

This is at the other extreme of the communication spectrum. Whereas passivity is the weakest form of communicating a message, aggression is extremely strong and usually too much in most circumstances. A person exhibiting aggressive behaviour does not acknowledge the rights and opinions of others and shows little or no respect for their workload or situation. Aggressive people view most communications as a battle to be won and they are in little doubt as to who is going to win it. Their style of communication is often intimidating, raising their voice and using threatening body language to get what they want at the expense of other people. The aggressive influencing style may yield short-term results through intimidation of others, but it is not a sustainable strategy in the longer term. Even the most passive people will eventually find a way to subvert the aggressive individual who will find themselves increasingly isolated.

What does it mean to be assertive?

Assertiveness is the middle ground between aggression and passivity. Assertive people stand up for themselves whilst respecting the rights and opinions of other people. They are not out to win a battle. They seek agreement and compromise in order for all parties to get what they want and emerge with a winning solution. Assertive people are very comfortable with their emotions both negative and positive and are able to express them accordingly. An assertive person could easily explain to another why they could not commit to another piece of work and would happily give the reasons why without feeling embarrassed or guilty. Assertive people know what they want and they understand their responsibilities. They are able to negotiate and persuade others when challenged to do something they believe to be inappropriate. To be assertive does not mean being rude or overly forceful. It means being clear and concise and, in the context of time management, being confident enough to own your refusal.

When you have become organised and put your priorities in order you will not want the situation to re-occur. Adopting an assertive style of communication will assist you in delegating certain tasks to other people and refusing certain requests because you need some time to focus on your priority projects.

Learning to be assertive

It is possible to learn assertive behaviours and like any new skill it will require practice. Success will not happen overnight! Even when you improve your assertiveness skills you will still encounter certain people or situations which undermine your confidence. There will always be times when it is more difficult to say no or to reach a compromise with someone. In these situations it is common to lose one's temper or to resentfully give in to the request. Either way the outcome is not good for either party. Lack of assertiveness over the long term can lead to loss of self-confidence and a lowering of self-esteem. It is possible to descend into a negative spiral, giving in to all demands and feeling worse and worse about doing so.

The best way to learn assertive behaviour is to take small steps. Practise saying no with friends and start to refuse minor requests, which have little impact on your working life. You may experience difficulties at first but this is a natural part of the process of developing a new habit.

Keep your objectives in your wallet or in the top drawer of your desk. Stick them on the wall in front of you. It doesn't matter where, as long as you keep them in sight. Print out a copy of your weekly schedule and have constant sight of that also. These reminders of your commitments will help you say yes to your own work and no to the work of other people.

Be convincing

Assertiveness refers to the strength of our communication. Many doctors find that even when they have said no, other people continue to challenge them and will not take no for an answer. This common reaction could be one of two factors. Either the requester is very aggressive in their behaviour and approach and is seeking to overwhelm and intimidate the other person, or the person saying no is not convincing enough.

When we communicate, in a face to face situation, there are 3 elements to the communication. Although the words we speak are very important, particularly in the context of assertiveness, they are not enough to convince someone. In terms of their influential impact they are very insignificant which may surprise some readers of this book. We place a lot of emphasis on our words and yet they may not be enough.

The second element of the communication is the voice and how it is used. This includes the tone, the pitch, the volume and the speed at which the words are spoken. The voice has a lot more influence than the spoken word when it comes to convincing others that you mean what you say. So, when you make a refusal to someone else's request, you have to sound convincing. If any doubt, hesitancy or anxiety is evident in your voice, the other person will continue to challenge you because they will realise that eventually you will give in. The prolonged exchange often does lead to anxiety and stress and the person attempting assertiveness will ultimately concede. Do not allow these indicators to show. If you are softly spoken, inject some volume into your voice. If your voice lacks conviction, introduce a tone of authority. Do not speak too quickly or too slowly. Find the balance so that you can speak with clarity and conviction. Make sure that when you do speak you are concise and not over talking, due to your anxiety.

The third element is the one which carries the largest amount of influence on another person, in a face to face exchange. This element relates to your body language. If you want someone to accept your refusal (or if you want someone to carry out your delegated task) then your words, voice and body language have to be aligned and convey the same meaning.

Your body language is so influential it is worth paying the closest attention to this element. Make sure that your stance is open. Folded arms or clenched hands could indicate a lack of openness and honesty. Clenched hands, in particular, could give the impression of anxiety. Make full eye contact when you are saying no or asking a colleague to do some work for you. Good eye contact indicates self-confidence and assertiveness. It demonstrates to others that you are not afraid to assert your rights and you do not feel guilty about doing so. Failure to do so creates the impression that you are uncomfortable with what you are saying and do not mean a word of it. This is often when the other person will start to challenge you in the hope of overwhelming you and forcing you to give way to their demands. They may not always do this aggressively. Some people will resort to charm and flattery and appeal to your heroic side. They will tell you that you are the only person in the team who does the task well enough. They may say that you are the only person they trust to do the job properly. Or they may praise your reliability and thank you for your commitment. Do not be fooled. Return to the safety of your objectives and weekly schedule. Before committing to anything, make sure that you really have got some time to spare. If you have not, it will help your assertive statements because you will be telling the truth and will feel less guilty as a result. The other person will hear that truth in your voice and will likely accept what you say.

Finally, be careful of giveaway facial expressions. If, when saying no, you grimace or deploy some other nervous facial gesture you are again demonstrating what you really feel on the inside. It is a clear invitation to the other person to try again as you are communicating an incongruent message. Although you may be saying no to someone, what you are really saying is, 'I do not believe in what I am saying so please ask me again and this time I will say yes.'

Time management tip

The unspoken message is much more powerful than the spoken word.

Putting the three elements together

Do not say 'maybe' when you mean no. The requester will believe that you are considering accepting and may keep trying to persuade you or pressurise you. If you want to say no you must do so. If that is too much too soon for you, then ask for some time to consider the request. Perhaps you need to check your weekly schedule? That is a genuine reason and shows you to be an organised person with definite commitments. Make sure you give a timeframe by when you will let the other person know and keep to that agreement.

Smile when you offer your refusal. Not many people will be offended by a refusal if it is said in a pleasant and factual manner. Make sure your voice carries a friendly but decisive tone. You are not engaged in a power struggle, even if an aggressive person wants you to be. You are simply stating the truth that, regrettably, you do not have time at the moment.

Example:

Time management tip

Putting the communication together for a congruent message

Words:	No I'm sorry I can't help, I have to finish this report this afternoon.
Voice:	Neutral tone of voice Clear, calm Moderate volume Moderate but decisive pace
Body Language	Full eye contact Smile (if appropriate) Open arms/hands (no nervous gestures)

Remove passive phrases from your language. If you are a habitual user of, 'is that okay?' or 'would you mind?' make a conscious effort to eliminate these from your repertoire! These seemingly innocent and polite words are actually subliminal requests for permission. If you manage to express your refusal, tagging on 'is that okay?' at the end will completely undermine your assertiveness. You hand the power back to the requester and all your efforts are wasted. When you feel those words about to emerge, just pause and then continue with the assertive part of the statement. Again, this will feel very odd at first but you will get used to it and you will be pleased with the results.

Another useful assertiveness technique is called the 'broken record'. Whilst many people will accept your refusal and think none the worse of you, there are some people who really do not want to take no for an answer. This technique is especially useful for them. As the name of the technique would imply you need to become a broken record and repeat yourself every time the other person challenges you. They want you to give into their demand. All you have to do is keep saying no and give your reasons in different ways. Begin with 'no' and take it from there:

No, I am not available tomorrow.

No, I am sorry but tomorrow is fully booked.

No, I'm not around tomorrow but I am available on Friday morning.

No I don't have any free time tomorrow.

Maintain full eye contact so that the subliminal message indicates you are speaking honestly and do not fold your arms, making you appear defensive. Keep your voice neutral and remove any petulant or angry tones. If you are truly being assertive you will remember that refusing does not involve being rude and you will respect their right to ask as well as your own right to refuse.

Negotiate to no

If saying the word 'no' really is too much for you, it is perfectly acceptable to negotiate an alternative. This is still refusing, but this time you are offering a solution, another aspect of being assertive.

Below are some examples of assertive statements which will be built, step by step, into an assertive negotiation. If you remember, assertiveness is about standing up for your rights whilst respecting the right of others. Some people like to begin their assertive statement by acknowledging the rights of the other person:

I understand the pressure you are under...........

I appreciate we are all busy at the moment.............

I realise you need to get this done...............

It is appropriate to follow this acknowledgement with your rebuttal. Use 'I' statements to indicate that you own your refusal:

.... but I'm sorry I cannot help you today..........

.... but I need you to do this extra task for me.........

.... but I am already fully committed this week...........

If you feel confident enough, you can stop talking at this point. You have respectfully acknowledged the other person's predicament but you have still said no, for whatever reason. You could leave it at that, but if it sounds too harsh, abrupt or rude to you, then you may want to offer an alternative. By doing so you are offering a solution, something that is typical of the assertive approach.

.... but I could come in early tomorrow if that would help.

.... I could help out next month.

.... I know that Jane has some spare time. Perhaps she could help you today?

To be assertive it would be ideal to begin your refusal with the word no. However, when you are starting out, you may want to try some gentler ways of getting to your refusal:

I'm sorry, but..........

I would like to, but............

I'm afraid that........

Unfortunately I won't be able to............

Saying no to seniors

For many doctors the idea of saying no to a senior colleague is unthinkable and impossible. It is true to say that it is never easy and can create the usual fears around saying no. You have to use your judgement. If you genuinely believe it would be a bad career move for you then you will have to delegate more of your work to other people or negotiate some extended deadlines.

Before you resort to this it is probably worth exploring some alternative options. If your senior gives you extra work, on the odd occasion, you should now have enough room in your weekly schedule to accommodate this. (Remember to leave some space for unexpected events and requests.) However, if the extra work is being delegated to you on a regular basis and it has nothing to do with your objectives, then it is definitely worth a discussion.

Often these situations arise due to a lack of clarity on both sides. Many junior doctors are unsure of what is expected of them but they do not like to ask, fearing that they should already know. If this describes you, put this conversation in the context of your improved time management. If you are to organise yourself more effectively, something your senior will welcome, then it is imperative that you discuss and agree your role, your workload and your objectives. You never know, your senior colleague may welcome the discussion too, as it gives them the opportunity to clarify your role and responsibilities.

Key items to agree

- Your responsibilities
- Your objectives
- Acceptable overtime
- Any support you require for particular projects
- All deadlines

Having agreed the above, if your senior persists in giving you work that has nothing to do with your objectives you can confidently discuss this issue. Inform your consultant or senior colleague that you are unable to concentrate on your objectives because of the additional work. Gain agreement that one or more of your objectives can be put to one side in favour of the new work. As long as you both agree there should be no problem with your performance or your appraisal. You may want to get the agreement in writing.

Approach this situation in a positive way. Accept some work from your senior when it is possible for you to do so. If it really is not possible, demonstrate this by sharing your weekly schedule. You will be judged far more harshly on your poor performance (brought on by an inability to say no to extra work or duties) than by the fact you have had to say no occasionally. If people see your planned work they will respect your refusal because they will understand it. Alternatively your senior may decide that an activity you had planned for that week can be dropped in favour of the new piece of work. As long as the decision has been made by them, then this should present no problems for you. Often your senior will find someone else to do that piece of work you had planned in order to free your time. There are many options available to you than just accepting the demands of a higher ranking colleague.

Double check the deadline

Rather like the section on negotiating above, it is always worth challenging your assumptions about when some work is due. Particularly where your senior is concerned, it is common practice to assume that, whatever their request, the work has to be done immediately. If you do not find out you will never know if your assumption is true. Some doctors have found that, when asked if they could defer the work to another day, agreement was immediately forthcoming. However, had they not queried the assumed deadline, the option of another day would not have been offered. So, be assertive and find out the true deadline for the work.

Key things to ascertain:

- Does it have to be done today?
- Can it wait until another day?
- Can anyone else do it who can meet the deadline?
- Can it be done tomorrow even if that means coming in early?

As you can see this is just another aspect of negotiating. If your week is planned properly you may well avoid saying no by finding out that the deadline is not immediate and that you have some spare capacity later in the week. If you are able to help and you feel it is an acceptable and fair request, do so, as you are part of a busy team and it is essential that you provide your support where you can for the sake of your patients.

Saying no to patients

This can be even harder for doctors than saying no to their senior colleague. Patients can be talkative whether they are in a hospital bed or in a General Practitioner's surgery. Clinics over-run and lists are not dealt with efficiently because doctors feel unable to leave their patients. This inability to take control of the situation will greatly undermine your time management techniques. Even if you have a plan you will not be able to stick to it if you allow your patients to continue talking. However, many doctors struggle to find a way of communicating this as they feel guilty and worry that they will appear abrupt or uncaring.

Try thinking of the situation differently. An effective doctor, who makes decisions and remains focused on his or her commitments, will be a far safer doctor and will provide better patient care. Learn to set expectations. Give your patients an idea of how long they have to speak:

In the ten minutes we have together..................

Unfortunately we don't have long, so let's start with....................

This does not make you uncaring. It makes you effective as you have many patients who need your care and attention. If a patient does not want to stop talking you can offer to return at a later time, while explaining that you have to continue your ward round or clinic or that you have a lot of patients to see in the waiting room. Be courteous and kind but be firm.

Exercise

Practise being assertive.

Begin by standing in front of a mirror and consciously controlling your body language. Keep your arms by your side, initially and say aloud some of the phrases given in this chapter. It is important that you hear yourself being assertive so that you can become accustomed to it.

Ensure that your voice carries authority. Be pleasant but firm and be clear and concise.

Practise some assertive phrases on friends and get feedback on how convincing you are. Remember that the 3 elements of your communication must all be giving the same signals so that other people accept your refusal or alternative option.

Set yourself a personal objective of being assertive once a week. If you are successful, increase this gradually until you are being assertive once a day. This could mean making a decision and acting upon it or it could mean talking to colleagues or patients.

Summary

- People make assumptions about what others will think of them if they say no. These are misconceptions.

- Childhood conditioning and some cultures make us believe that is wrong to say no. However, it is possible to learn how to say no without causing offence to others.

- The three influencing styles are passivity, assertiveness and aggression. For effective time management it is essential to be assertive.

- Assertiveness enables you to stand up for your rights whilst not damaging the rights of others. This means you can offer compromises, alternative solutions and explain why you are unable to commit to extra work. Assertiveness means telling the truth.

- If saying no is too much, it is possible to negotiate an alternative option. This may mean you have still said no or it may mean that you agree to do the work on your own terms, according to your schedule.

- If your senior colleague is delegating too much on a regular basis, discuss and agree your role, responsibilities and duties and if your objectives have changed, get this in writing.

- Double check all deadlines in case you have incorrectly assumed that a task is urgent. Challenging a deadline often leads to clarity of expectations.

Chapter 11　The final act – developing the habit of personal effectiveness

Aims & objectives

In this chapter you will:

- Realise the importance of maintaining your system of prioritising

- Develop better systems to deal with the day-to-day flow of paper, e-mails and telephone calls

- Understand why meetings can be such time wasters

- Learn how to chair meetings effectively

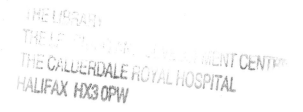

Becoming personally effective

Good time management must be applied to all your communication systems. In order to remain focused on your priorities, you need to develop ways of dealing with your paperwork, your e-mails, telephone calls and meetings you attend. In order to become personally effective, you must increase your organisational skills and complete your essential activities as well as delivering the best possible service to your patients. A disorganised doctor cannot provide this.

It is worth remembering the impression you may be giving your patients. Your internal emotions are easily conveyed to other people through your body language and demeanour. If you are stressed how do you think this will affect your patients? Perhaps they may doubt your abilities to treat them properly. Develop an air of calm control and systematically work your way through your daily commitments as you have planned them. Be pleasant but firm with your colleagues and patients alike. Remember your responsibilities and execute them.

Your aim, having become organised, must be to stay that way. Unless you apply a similar discipline towards all the facets of a working day, you will be unable to focus on your essential and immediate priorities. Your challenge is to maintain your new methods. You must prevent a return to dealing with other people's requests and the escapist activities which relieve your stress. Applying an organised approach to information overload via e-mails, paperwork and telephones, will enable you to do this. Although this book has extensively covered the skills you need, here is a summary of what you need to do on a weekly basis in order to remain organised.

The key elements of personal effectiveness

- Keep your objectives visible.

- Prioritise your activities each week (not each day).

- Spend most of your time on essential activities and do not defer them until the deadline forces you into frenetic action.

- Break your tasks into activities.

- Schedule a realistic amount of activities into your diary.

- Leave time in your daily schedule for interruptions and unexpected events.

- Schedule some one-to-one meetings to review complex delegated tasks. (Remember you need to stay informed.)

- Address any concerns in these meetings. Give feedback in the form of constructive comments or offer your praise and support.

- If you are a junior doctor, do most of the above and delegate what you can or negotiate more effectively so that you can meet your priorities.

Develop better systems

Part of your overall effectiveness involves developing systems to deal with everyday issues, such as paperwork and all forms of communication, such as e-mails and telephone calls. Doctors who manage their time well know what to do with every piece of paper that crosses their desk each day. They create a system for reading and dealing with their e-mail and they even develop ways of coping with telephone calls. With the same focus and determination you have begun to apply to your tasks and activities, you must now do the same for all other areas of your working life if you want to support your new system of prioritising. Even meetings can be streamlined or run more efficiently to release more time to focus on your important activities. This chapter explores some options for improving your efficiency and you can use these as a starting point for developing your own style. As long as the outcome is achieved, that of eliminating time-wasting actions, it does not really matter which method you develop.

Dealing with the paperwork

Why reduce your paperwork?

Although apparently an obvious question it is a message worth re-iterating in the context of time management. All doctors work long hours, in often pressurised conditions and it is easy to leave the filing for another day.

As you well know, one day rushes into another and soon you have an unmanageable amount of paperwork on your desk, some of which may be essential to your working life.

This is a critical point and a huge incentive for becoming more organised. If it takes you a long time to locate important information, the impact on other people and processes could be significant. A reduction in your paperwork will actually improve communication in the team. You will be able to conduct better handovers with your colleagues if you can retrieve the information you need easily. If you are absent your colleagues need to be able to find relevant patient information. They cannot do their job successfully without it. Not only must patient notes be written up in a timely manner and not deferred until later in the week, your colleagues need to be able to access them when they need them. Poor time management often leads to delays in this area and frustration for the whole team. If you are a senior doctor, leading a team, this is even more important. Teams can only be empowered to make decisions when they have the necessary information available. It is your responsibility to ensure you provide that information or develop a system that everyone can use when sharing data. If you do not, you run the risk of nothing happening in your absence and your service to patients will be severely impaired.

What should you do with it?

Can you easily locate the documents you need whenever you need them? Or are you part of the majority who have so much paperwork that it takes a long time to find anything you want? You may have a filing tray or a set of three that stack on top of one another and yet still be unable to find what you want easily and efficiently. This is a frustrating position to be in but paperwork is something you cannot escape in medicine, even with the initiative to hold more records electronically.

What are your reasons for keeping paper?

Perhaps you need to read articles for your reference or interest but never quite have the time to read them. Numerous magazines pile up on your desk, or beneath your desk, but in reality it is unlikely you ever get around to reading them, particularly if the pile is growing. Having to read through the magazines again to find the article of interest is off-putting and the sheer volume of articles to read can be daunting. You may have decided that these articles will be useful for your specialty or general reference but how true is that in reality if you do not read them as they are published?

Many doctors simply do not know why they hang onto so much paper. In many cases they simply do not know what to do with it and leave it to sit in the in-tray or on their desk. Some doctors work on the premise that if no-one chases them up for a response the paper can eventually be disposed of. This method usually requires six months and ensures an untidy desk for that length of time. Other doctors throw away paper they do not know what to do with, again after a suitable period of holding time.

Are you a doctor that hoards all paper in the belief that it may be useful to you one day? You are not alone! Many doctors create whole filing systems around paperwork that they never refer to again but hold the belief that one day it may be of use. If you are like that, re-visit your reasoning. Examine the paper you kept six months ago for that reason and ask yourself if it has proved useful to you so far. If it has not done so yet, it is unlikely that it ever will. Be a bit tougher with yourself and get rid of superfluous paper that you know will not be useful to you in the future. You may be retaining some reports or letters in order to pass them on to a colleague. This is a valid reason as long as you do pass them on in a timely fashion.

Finally, you may be holding on to reference material in order to build a knowledge pool. Any information pertaining to your specialty may be kept for your own reference or for the team or departmental reference. This is an excellent reason for retaining the paperwork that arrives on your desk as long as the information is available as intended.

One area of paperwork that must be addressed quickly is the written complaint which is sometimes received from patients. You have little choice but to act on this type of letter quickly. Therefore, it is imperative that you have a system established that can deal with this. However, if it is possible to deal with complaints effectively, why not the other types of letters or reports? What is stopping you from imposing a similar strict response time on yourself for these types of correspondence?

Limit the time you spend searching for paper on your desk. Deal with items as soon as possible so that you can clear your desk and file or dispense with them by other means. If you do not apply the same focus and discipline to this area as you do to your activities, then you begin to undermine your own efforts at improved time management.

The choices for action

You have a number of options when deciding how best to handle your paperwork. It is likely that the most effective choice is to act on it so that it does not remain on your desk or in your filing tray for long.

However, it may be appropriate to action it via delegation and passing it to someone else for action. Letters which require a response should be passed to the secretarial team as soon as possible. Some reports could be actioned by a colleague perhaps. If someone else could, in theory, deal with that paperwork; do not hesitate to let them.

Another option is to file the paper but only do this if retaining the paper is necessary. Ensure that you have helpful filing systems which enable you to re-locate the item if you need it.

There is a strong possibility that you can throw away some of the paperwork on your desk. As mentioned previously, if you have not taken action on a report or reference material and months have passed, it is probably not worth keeping. If the magazines piling up under your desk have not been read the information contained within them may well be out of date by now. Be brutal and throw out those items you know you will never deal with and which do not require action.

Another choice is to deal with the paperwork at a future date. This is acceptable as long as you can find somewhere meaningful to store it for that interim period. Set up a system for pending items or those which need your eventual attention, which could be between the present and the next 6 months. Some doctors very successfully use a concertina folder which has at least 12 pockets, each labelled with the months of the year. Papers which require action at a point in the future get placed in the relevant month, remaining there until needed. This is a convenient way of filing necessary, but not immediate, pieces of work which can be retrieved effortlessly.

What must be retained?

It is common knowledge that financial records must be retained for a seven-year period but it is likely that the administration office will handle this. Some legal paperwork must also be kept, particularly anything pertaining to complaints. Patient records form the most obvious source of information which must be retained but again, it is to be hoped that each hospital has effective systems in place to hold this kind of information. Relating to your more personal paperwork which pieces of information do you feel you should retain? This does not refer to the 'just in case' type of reading material, but necessary day to day paperwork that it would be wrong to throw away. Take a good look at your desk and group together the paper you know you cannot afford to get rid of.

Clear the clutter

Just as you began to organise yourself by sorting all your outstanding actions into an order of priority, it would be useful to do the same with your paperwork. In order to become organised you need to deal with the situation as it exists now. Having identified the need to deal with your paperwork both in the short and longer term, here is a suggested solution to help you get started. One of your choices will be to throw out any paper that you do not need. If your hospital provides re-cycling bins, you may like to use them to dispose of your unwanted paper.

As part of your weekly scheduling, allocate as much time as you can, preferably 2 hours, to clearing your desk. If you cannot afford that much time, try scheduling a shorter amount of time but consider doing this more than once in the week. Aim for 2-3 opportunities to tackle the paperwork on your desk.

Your task is to deal with every single piece of paper currently on your desk and you have two main choices. You can either file it or throw it away. Have an empty bin liner with you before you start this exercise. You may be surprised at how much you can dispose of!

Remove all gadgets, toys, picture frames and other office equipment such as staplers and hole punchers. All loose pens must be gathered up and placed in a container such as a desk tidy or spare mug. The only thing on your desk apart from the paper should be three filing trays. If you do not have that number of trays, obtain them. You cannot achieve anything meaningful until you have them. You may want to label your trays with the following headings: Action, Pending and File.

Work through every piece of paper and assign it to one of the three trays or put it in your waste bag or recycling bin.

Action tray

For the pieces of paper you have assigned to *Action*, you then have to decide what action to take. For things which require fairly immediate action you can either do them yourself, provided you have allocated enough time, or you can delegate them.

Pending tray

The same choices apply here. Consider writing a date on the top of the paper to give you a sense of priority. When will that piece of paper be actioned? Do not leave things in this tray which will not be done in the current month. Move those longer term pieces of paper to your concertina file and keep this file in a three-drawer pedestal filing cabinet which sits beneath your desk. This may be another piece of office furniture you need to acquire. Regarding the paper you have allocated to *Pending*, you may decide to delegate some of these items too, in which case you must schedule a delegation meeting at the appropriate time.

File tray

Put anything here that you really cannot delegate or throw away and that you have decided you really must keep. Ensure that you have a proper filing system, or that it passes to the departmental filing system. If you are building a knowledge pool you may want a drawer which contains 26 hanging folders which are labelled A-Z. This makes it easy for you to file by topic heading. For other filing you may want to consider category headings such as Complaints, Reports, Audit, Research and so on. Choose the system that has the most meaning for you.

Maintaining a clear desk

As well as your filing tray system, telephone and computer, make sure you have your objectives on your desk. Some doctors keep paper diaries and put their objectives at the front so that they are always visible. You must keep connected with your motivation for effective time management and your objectives will help to provide this.

As part of your weekly priority scheduling, make sure that you include some time each week to deal with the filing. This would be a useful Friday activity and need not take long once you have become organised.

Schedule in a daily activity which deals with administration, so that you create time to deal with your *Action Now* items or have them ready for a delegation meeting. You will find it useful to start your day organising your paperwork so perhaps the initial 15 minutes of your day could begin this way?

Remember that the only paperwork on your desk should be that which has come out of your filing trays.

New paperwork

Now that you have a successful system for dealing with paperwork, apply it to all new paperwork that arrives. Simply decide whether it needs to be actioned now, later or needs filing.

Magazines

A quick way of reducing the pile of paper beneath (or on top of) your desk is to extract the article you wish to read and discard the rest of the magazine into your recycling bin. Place all the articles in one of your trays. When future publications arrive, put them in the *Pending* tray and when you have the time, skim through them and tear out any article you wish to keep for future reference. This method will keep your filing to a minimum and use up much less storage space.

If you commute to and from work on the train or bus, use this transition time to catch up with your article reading. When you use all the time available wisely it is surprising how much you can accomplish. Effective use of your time really is about making the best use of the time at your disposal. Commuting provides a wonderful opportunity for catching up with reading as well as replying to e-mails on an electronic organiser.

Coping with e-mails

E-mails have become part of our everyday life and whilst they were initially deemed as an aid to improved communication, for many they have become a burden. As with paperwork, it would be useful to develop a system for dealing with the amount of e-mails you receive each day. Ideally you should create designated times for reading your e-mails. No doctor has the luxury of remaining behind a desk all day, monitoring and replying to e-mails as they arrive. That habit, in itself, can be distracting and destructive. With ward rounds and clinics to run it is almost easier for doctors to allocate set times for e-mail. First thing in the morning, lunchtimes and towards the end of the day are favoured times for many doctors. You should avoid spending more than three occasions attending to your inbox. Three visits should ensure you stay on top of incoming correspondence and systems similar to your paperwork can be created.

Do not waste time and create more paper by printing your e-mails. Create folders in your e-mail system and detach documents and spreadsheets and file electronically. There is nothing to stop you creating an *Action* and *Pending* folder within your e-mail account, if you wish.

If you receive jokes on e-mail or chain e-mails from colleagues and friends, let it be known that you no longer wish to be included. Remove yourself from superfluous e-mail distribution lists. Some organisations include 'ACTION REQUIRED' notifications in the subject of their e-mail, indicating to colleagues which e-mails require immediate attention. Could you introduce this into your hospital?

If you are copied on e-mails for information purposes, but do not need to be, get yourself removed from carbon copy lists or explain to the regular distributors of these e-mails that you do not need to be included. Minimise your e-mails as much as you can and deal with the rest in a controlled and planned manner.

The telephone

As was revealed in the chapter on setting priorities, some doctors allow a ringing telephone to become a method for prioritisation. As soon as one starts ringing, they stop whatever they are working on and answer it. This can be fatal to the successful completion of a planned task. You do not know who may be at the end of the telephone or how long the call will last. Even if the call is short, the interruption to your thought processes will take a few minutes to recover. Precious minutes are lost with every interruption.

If you have scheduled time to do something, switch on the voice-mail or message system on the telephone so that the call is automatically diverted to that service. Deal with the message only when you have completed your task.

Do the same with your mobile phone or handheld device. Switch them to the silent or vibrate option so that you are not disturbed when you need to concentrate, providing you are not on call.

If you need to make a call, plan carefully before you do so, so that you know what you want to say and stick to it. With any interaction, be it face-to-face or on the telephone, you should always plan your outcome. Why are you making the call? What do you want or need to achieve? If you start with the end in mind, you can plan more effectively for it. Decide upon the facts you need to include, or salient arguments you wish to use. Most importantly, consider what time you have available to make the call. Is it enough? If it is not, but you cannot extend the timeframe, prioritise what you want to say and cover the most salient points. This should help you avoid being sidetracked by the person to whom you are speaking.

For many doctors it is the patient telephone calls which are likely to take longer than expected. Many patients understandably need to talk and some doctors experience feelings of guilt when faced with closing the call before a patient is ready. If this reaction resonates with you remember that you have many patients who need you and it is acceptable to be empathetic whilst remaining assertive because the situation demands it. So, if a particular patient is known to be needy or who always prolongs the call, manage their expectations at the start. Here are some examples of assertive and expectation-setting phrases:

'I'm afraid I only have five minutes, but I wanted to tell you ...'

'I have to see another patient at 12pm but I am ringing to make another appointment for you next week. We can have a proper chat then.'

'I only have 10 minutes available so can you tell me briefly what the problem is?'

You are not being rude but you are being factual about how much time you have. Do not undermine yourself by then allowing the patient to talk indefinitely. Stick to the time you have stated. Apologise at the end of the call if you have to but try and end the call. You must strike a balance between concise and caring. Be firm with your time but caring towards your patients.

Meeting mania

Meetings are one of the biggest time wasters in modern working life. Many are held for the sake of it and many continue long after they have served their original purpose because they become part of the fabric of the working week and have become habitual. Some, however, are very useful and serve as an efficient means of conveying information to a large group of people. Meetings cannot be eliminated but perhaps they can be reduced or chaired more effectively in order to maximise their usefulness for all attendees. In medicine, the practice of holding team meetings can be problematical for some attendees, even though the idea is well intentioned. For example, non-clinical team members can become very bored when the majority of the agenda concerns topics they know little about and cannot follow. Yet they are expected to sit through long meetings and listen to clinical discussions that probably do not affect them. Perhaps they could be spending that time more effectively? As a doctor, consider how you could get the information to the whole team without them having to be present? If you did want them to attend, could non-clinical agenda items be dealt with first and then the non-clinical staff could be released to get on with their priorities?

Why are meetings such time wasters?

Some meetings do not start on time due to the late arrival of certain individuals. Rather than commencing without them, many chairmen or women would prefer to wait, believing that the meeting would only have to re-start once everyone was in attendance.

Many meetings are not chaired effectively and if there are a number of strong personalities present, it can be difficult to stick to the agenda.

Some individuals can be difficult to quieten and it is easy to see how some meetings descend into little more than heated debate. With so many people wanting to be heard and a weak Chair unable to control the situation, these types of meetings take far longer than they should.

The secrets of efficient meetings

Establish who needs to attend. If you are chairing the meeting and decide that all the team should be present, consider the advice given previously and think about beginning with non-clinical items and allowing administrative staff the option of leaving after those items have been discussed and actioned.

Start the meeting on time and make it clear to everyone that if they are late they will miss what has been discussed.

If you are in the position of Chair use your assertiveness skills and ensure that everyone follows the agenda and does not introduce other topics. If they do, question the relevance of the question or debate and remind everyone of the agenda item they are meant to be discussing.

Ensure that any actions arising are allocated clearly and that the individuals concerned understand the action they have been given. Agree deadlines for all actions and follow them up after the meeting so that all team members take their tasks seriously.

Circulate the minutes of the meeting in a timely fashion, preferably the same day. This will provide useful information for anyone not in attendance or latecomers who may have missed the beginning. If appropriate, help the minute-taker by advising him or her which items to record. When long discussions ensue it can be difficult for someone to judge accurately. As Chair, you should decide which points are pertinent to capture. This will include all actions.

As a meeting attendee

Review all the meetings you currently attend and decide whether you really do need to be there. Could you obtain all the information you need from reading a copy of the minutes? If the answer is yes then consider removing the meeting from your diary. If you need agreement from your senior then discuss it with them. Give your reasons and explain that you can keep up-to-date via the minutes.

An alternative to this approach would be to delegate your attendance. Perhaps a colleague in the team, or if you are senior, one of your junior team members, could attend in your place? You can save useful time by having a shorter summary meeting with that individual afterwards.

Negotiate with the Chairman your requirement to leave after certain agenda topics have been discussed. This approach works well for many doctors.

Exercise

Review how you deal with all your systems:

Start by clearing the clutter from your desk. Follow the advice given in this chapter and see how much paper you can reduce or eliminate.

Decide how you want to manage your e-mails and practise scheduling a regular time for reading them. Make this part of your weekly planning process.

Plan one telephone call in advance. Decide upon your outcome and write down, in bullet point format, what you need to say. Decide how long you wish to spend on the call and practise starting the conversation with a sentence that sets the right expectations. Make the call and see if you can implement your plan.

Review your meetings and calculate how much time they collectively take from your working week. If appropriate, decide which meetings you can drop and consider negotiating shorter attendance times with your Chairperson.

If you are the Chair, consider what ways you could run the meeting more effectively so that it makes the best use of everyone's time.

Summary

- It is essential to be as disciplined in all work related systems as with your system of prioritising tasks and activities.

- Paperwork must be dealt with as quickly as possible, even if that means just making a decision about into which filing tray it is placed.

- Do not be tempted to review your e-mail inbox throughout the day. Allocate time in your weekly planning and view the reading of e-mails as a task. It is advisable to schedule this task twice or three times during each working day.

- If you are working on a specific priority, ensure that your telephone does not distract you. Switch mobiles to the 'silent' option or desk telephones to the messaging service.

- Most meetings are a threat to successful time management because they do not start on time and do not stick to the agenda. Many over-run and may not even serve their purpose.

- Consider requesting the minutes of some meetings as a substitute for being there.

- If you chair meetings, being assertive will be your greatest asset. Everyone has given up their time to attend, so ensure that time is used wisely. Quieten down the strong, talkative individuals, ensure everyone has a chance to speak if they need to and above all, keep the meeting on track by adhering to the agenda.

Chapter 12 Get a life!

Aims & objectives

In this chapter you will:

- Learn the importance of developing a work/life balance
- Develop a system for good life management
- Identify your life roles
- Set some goals in your personal life
- Learn how to lead a fulfilling life by taking action and stop procrastination

There is more to life than work

Time management tip

Successful time managers develop and maintain a good work/life balance.

Doctors who are successful at managing their time pay equal attention to their personal life, including leisure time. They understand that work cannot be everything in itself. Work can only be part of a satisfying life in that it provides a fulfilling career but cannot be enough to satisfy all human needs.

However, doctors appear to lose sight of this fact more rapidly than other professions. The long hours and pressurised environment of medicine isolate many clinicians to the point where all hobbies and interests are abandoned. Personal relationships and family life can also be significantly affected. Female clinicians tell of the struggle to maintain the household and the needs of their children when they return from work. Many feel they are unable to spend proper time with their children and some speak of their distress when they become aware that, due to fatigue, all they do is shout at them. Whatever the personal situation, whenever work begins to dominate life, the individual is entering into dangerous territory.

This book has devoted itself to introducing options for improvement of your time management skills in the workplace. Why not transfer these strategies for success into your personal life? If you could apply the same focus and attention to other areas of your life, you might be able to even out any imbalances. The impact on your long-term well-being would be significant.

Why is work/life balance important?

According to The Mental Health Foundation, a leading UK charity that pioneers new ways of looking at mental health and has carried out extensive research during the last sixty years, the pressure of an increasingly demanding work culture in the UK is perhaps the biggest and most pressing challenge to the mental health of the general population. People

146 Effective Time Management Skills for Doctors

need other elements in their life, such as exercise, family relationships and outside interests. When these are neglected, due to the demands of work, the cumulative effect may cause some people to lose their mental resilience and lead to a lowering of resistance to stress.

It is estimated that nearly three in every ten employees will experience a mental health problem in any one year. However the recent and dramatic rise in Britain's working hours would suggest this is likely to increase. It is hoped that the European Working Time Directive will help to control this within medicine.

Life management

Do any of the following sound familiar?

> 'There aren't enough hours in the day.'
>
> 'All I think about is work, even when I'm at home.'
>
> 'I can't afford to switch off.'
>
> 'I'd like to catch up with friends, but there's never enough time.'

If you have ever found yourself thinking or saying this to other people, you may be in danger of focusing too much on work and neglecting your personal life. You may need to spend some time clarifying what you want to achieve or accomplish in each of the various areas of your life. It may also help you to identify your life roles. Perhaps you spend too much time being a clinician and not enough time being a parent or spouse. If this could be true for you, the sooner you deal with the situation the better. Any imbalances will leave you feeling stressed and out of control. You always have a choice. You can waste the time you have engaging in trivial activities or putting things off until another day or you can focus on meaningful and rewarding activities. As you can see, the same rules apply to home life as much as they do in your career. As much as possible, fill your life with worthwhile activities. The time you are granted ticks away no matter what you do with it. It would be a shame to have such a narrow focus, when you could be realising your potential and enjoying a full and varied life. How much better it would be if you were a doctor who enjoys your work and could retain an objective outlook on life. It would be helpful for you to remember that there is more to you than medicine. The first step to re-engaging with your true self is to identify your life roles.

Identifying your life roles

By identifying your life roles you are creating a variety of perspectives from which to examine your life and ensure that it carries the balance you need to live a fulfilling existence. For example, you may be a doctor, advisor, colleague, parent, son, daughter, sibling, school governor, charity worker, church-goer, cricket-team member, mentor and so on. Using the grid below, identify the various roles you fulfil in your life.

1.	
2.	
3.	
4.	
5.	
6.	
7.	

Figure 12.1 Life roles grid

Notice that seven categories have been allocated in the grid above. This is to remind you that any more might become unmanageable. The purpose of this exercise is to show that all parts of your life are inter-connected. Although you have been asked to categorise your life into roles, it is with the intention of helping you realise the impact on each area when you focus too much time on one. Your aim is always to integrate all the aspects and roles of your life. When planning your weekly schedule remember to include all your 'role' commitments. Make time for everything you need to fulfil, or be, for other people. If you want to read a bedtime story for your children once a week, schedule it in and stick to it.

How do you spend your time?

Just as you did with work, you will find it useful to set some personal objectives for the various non-working areas of your life. This is an effective technique used in life coaching as it enables individuals to quickly identify the areas of neglect and then to set some outcomes for improvement. You are going to complete what is called *the circle of life.*

Draw yourself a circle with a maximum of seven segments. Give each segment a title, pertaining to an area of your life. For example, Friends & Family could be one section; Health & Fitness might be another. Other examples include: Relaxation, Personal Development, Career, Church, Charities, Society or Environment. Choose the headings that are appropriate to your life and interests.

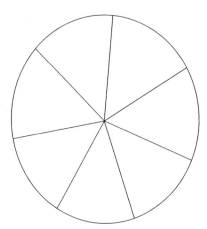

Figure 12.2 Circle of life

Now rate each segment out of ten. If you are very satisfied with a particular area of your life you will rate it nine or ten out of ten. If there are areas of your life where you have not accomplished what you want or it is not bringing you the satisfaction you hoped for, give it a lower rating.

Once you have given each area of your life a mark out of ten, focus on the segments which score less than seven out of ten. These areas are in need of your attention. Of each area in need of attention, ask yourself:

'How much time am I spending on this area of my life?'

'How much time do I want to be spending?'

'What do I need to do to improve this area of my life?'

Setting objectives

Ideally you should set some objectives for every area of your life that you have included in your wheel. At the very least you need to set some in the areas which were low scoring. You can see how the principles of time management at work apply equally well in your personal life. Setting outcomes in each *circle of life* area enables you to focus on parts of your life which may have been neglected until now. Perhaps you are feeling out of shape and wish to regain former fitness levels or lose some weight. Identifying and writing down a positive goal will help you achieve it, far more than wishful thinking. Make the commitment to spend more time on non-working activities and you will soon achieve a more balanced lifestyle and the inevitable peace of mind which goes with it. Many doctors set outcomes in the area of Family due to a prevailing desire to spend more quality time with the significant people in their lives.

Keep them SMART

Remember to shape your objectives following the SMART acronym. All your goals or objectives must be specific, measurable, achievable, realistic and time-framed.

Aim for balance

For those who experience difficulties or disappointments in their personal life, retreating into a world of work can often seem like the easiest option. Workaholics are usually individuals who procrastinate in other areas of their life. They escape into work, using it as an excuse not to deal with personal issues. However, this can seriously undermine their ability to be effective in their work role as their stress levels start to build due to some source of dissatisfaction. A balance must be struck if an individual is to maintain a sense of perspective and achieve an all-round sense of well-being. You will see similar patterns of behaviour arising in your personal life. Perhaps you struggle to say no to certain people or requests for favours. However, the rules remain the same.

You must learn to say no to the non-rewarding actions that fill your personal life. You must avoid procrastination and get on with the day to day obligations. If you do not, they will simply accumulate as your work commitments do when they are left unattended. Your mind will not let go of them until they are complete and so, yet again, you will be burdened by a sense of guilt or that feeling that you should have done something by now. You only have one life so deal with your commitments and then you are free to enjoy the time that is left each day.

Make a conscious effort to decide how much of your time you wish to spend on each segment of your *circle of life*. Work in percentages and if you find the time you would like to spend exceeds one hundred percent in total, be ruthless and make reductions in some areas. Be even more disciplined about saying no to things in your personal life that you really do not want to waste time on. Now you have a real motive because you have chosen to increase the amount of time you spend in each area of your life.

Experience a little déjà vu

It is important that you apply the same principles of time management to both your professional and personal life. This final chapter is about integrating all aspects of your life and putting you back in control. So the next steps may start to sound familiar. If you feel confident about the techniques described earlier in the book and are happy to implement them in your personal life, there is no need for you to read any more. If, however, you would like some guidance to get you started, the remainder of this chapter will show you how to sort out time management issues in the rest of your life and leave you ready to maintain your newly organised systems by implementing the techniques on a week by week basis.

Gather up your outstanding actions

There are probably a few things in your personal life that you have not had the time to deal with yet. Perhaps some of them are a bit complicated or require effort and it seems too much to get started. Here is a list of typical examples:

- Renew your passport
- Replace a lost or stolen driving licence
- Pay the gas bill
- Buy a birthday card
- Book a caterer for a forthcoming party
- Sign up for an exercise class
- Exercise daily
- Clear out the loft
- Tidy the garage
- Prune the garden plants
- Complete your dissertation
- Book the car in for a service
- Create new filing systems for your home study
- Complete some pre-course work for a training course

If you have many outstanding tasks, it may help you to categorise them into your *circle of life* segments. You can write each task in the appropriate segment which will give you an idea of how much you have to do in each area. If you do not have too many commitments awaiting your attention you may be able to schedule them into your diary immediately.

Viewing your commitments through the *circle of life* method does allow you to see which parts of your life you have been neglecting. When deciding upon a set of priorities, you can either choose to reduce a segment of your life which has many obligations listed within it, or you can decide which area of your life is the most important to you right now and deal with the actions within that.

It is also a useful way of helping you reflect upon your life and how you have been living it. When you review your actions, do you think you are repeating the same mistakes at home as at work? Are there people that you should be saying no to, but find yourself giving in? This may be true of your Friends and Family category, if you have one. It can be a lot harder to say no to a relative than a colleague. Friends often ask for favours but can you afford to say yes? The *circle of life* gives you the opportunity to see how many obligations you are accumulating and will help to reveal their source.

Perhaps it is time to re-focus. Think about the objectives you have set in each part of your life and remember your roles. What should you be spending time on and with whom? Put the things which are important to you first and start saying no more often to the things which you do not want to do or cannot spare the time to do. Be as clear about what you want to achieve in your home life as you are now in your working life.

An alternative option to help you prioritise is to use the mind map system. You can review the whole of your *circle of life* and decide which actions really must be done during the forthcoming week. In other words, what is important to you and how quickly must it be done? The renewal of a passport becomes very important and of the highest priority when a holiday is looming.

Next, turn your attention to the actions which are still important to you but can be scheduled for a later date. If the party is in September and the current month is April, perhaps a discussion or meeting with the caterers can wait until July? Again, do not under-estimate how long things can take. If you think a meeting in September would suffice you will suffer a disappointment. Events such as parties require a good deal of notice so err on the side of caution and plan ahead. The point is, the meeting can be planned and scheduled in advance if you take action on it now and do not put it off.

Turning to the third mind map, there may even be commitments which can be delegated to someone else! Perhaps it is your turn to ask for a favour from a friend or family member. Now that you have set some objectives it will be easier for you to say no to certain requests in future.

Resolve the immediate crisis

Before you can conduct the whole of your life in an organised manner, you must deal with the immediate list of outstanding actions, using the methods outlined above.

Having shaped your tasks into some sort of priority, it is imperative that you schedule some into your diary for the coming week. Remember not to over-estimate how much you can achieve, so limit yourself to the accomplishment of one or two tasks, depending upon their size and how much time you realistically need. If the tasks are relatively short you may want to schedule one more, but do not overload yourself by trying to complete everything in one week.

If the tasks are complex and time-consuming, see if you can break them down into smaller chunks of activity. Schedule some shorter activities into your weekly diary so that you have at least started to deal with the items you may have been resisting. Repeat this process each week until your list of outstanding commitments related to your personal life has been dealt with.

Ongoing success

This really is the final piece of the puzzle. It is one thing to get yourself out of a chaotic situation at work and at home but it is just as important to maintain that state of orderly calm. There will, of course, be times when your well-practised habit of scheduling each week may not happen, but if you start to feel out of control, return to the basics of this book and calmly review your priorities and deal with the most important. Do not be too hard on yourself if things slip occasionally. As long as you have the strategies to get back on track as soon as things calm down, you will be fine. Do not panic. Go back to the techniques which work for you and deploy them. For the majority of your time you do want to aim for a calm maintenance of your systems. This should be relatively easy to do once you have cleared the clutter in both your professional and personal life.

The idea now is to merge the two distinct areas of your life so that they are fully integrated. Bring your work and life together because continued compartmentalising can throw your life out of balance again and encourage you back into workaholic tendencies. Include a Work and Career segment into your *circle of life* which will help with the integration process. Here are some useful reminders to help you maintain the positive habits of effective time management and effective life management:

Managing your life's priorities effectively

- Keep all your goals or objectives visible (work and life).

- Schedule all commitments on a weekly basis – fixed appointments, work activities and home life activities.

- Focus on the activities which are most important to you and either must be done in the coming week or can help you get ahead of your deadlines.

- Learn to plan ahead by scheduling small actions on a regular basis so that you are always making progress.

- Remember all your life roles and what you mean to the people in your life.

- Do not put off until a later day what you can usefully deal with today.

A word about relaxation

If it is not in your *circle of life* already, consider including a segment entitled Relaxation or 'Me Time'. Making the time to unwind is critical to your mental and emotional well-being. However, it is usually the element we neglect the most. If you know that you tend to neglect yourself because you are so busy being 'someone' for other people, it would be advisable for you to schedule some weekly form of relaxation, alongside your tasks. Set an objective for yourself in this area. Perhaps for an hour a week you are going to read a favourite piece of fiction or simply relax in the armchair whilst listening to some music. Perhaps once a month you are going to book a facial or a massage or visit the cinema. Having an objective like this will remind you to take care of yourself and, more importantly, will enable you to plan it into your diary of commitments. You will definitely reap the benefits.

Never feel guilty for taking care of yourself. You have earned it.

Exercise

Draw a *circle of life* and divide it into a maximum of seven areas. Give each area a title which pertains to your life. Ensure that it aligns with your roles in life.

Give each area a score out of ten in terms of your satisfaction with that part of your life. Is it how you want it to be? Does it fulfil you? Could there be room for improvement?

For areas which score seven or under, set some meaningful objectives which will help improve it until you are able to score it above seven in three, six or twelve months' time.

Each week remember to schedule into your diary a task or activity which moves you towards the fulfilment of your objectives.

Include an area which relates to your own well-being and relaxation time.

Summary

- Developing and maintaining a healthy work-life balance is imperative for good mental health.

- Defining a personal *circle of life* helps you plan and prioritise the activities for all aspects of your life.

- Identifying your life roles can help you see where, and with whom, you need to spend more time, (or less time).

- Setting goals in your personal life will help you focus and maintain your attention and stop you from spending too much time in one area.

- Getting on with your life is far more productive and fulfilling than putting things off.

- Procrastination may inhibit your true potential.

- Aim to integrate your career and home life so that you can experience a well rounded life and maintain a proper sense of perspective.

References

European Working Time Directive (1998, 2003)
www.dh.gov.uk and www.healthcareworkforce.nhs.uk

The Academy of Medical Royal Colleges and the NHS Institute for Innovation and Improvement, *Medical Leadership Competency Framework* (2008)
www.institute.nhs.uk
(Can download the 80 page document in PDF format from this website)

Mental Health Foundation
http://www.mentalhealth.org.uk/

Stephen Covey, *The 7 Habits of Highly Effective People* Simon and Schuster UK Ltd (2004)

General Medical Council, *Tomorrows Doctors* (1993, 2003)
http://www.gmc-uk.org/education/undergraduate/undergraduate_policy/tomorrows_doctors.asp

Workforce Review Team (1999)
http://www.wrt.nhs.uk/

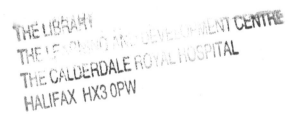

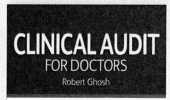
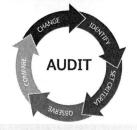

More Titles in the Progressing Your Medical Career Series

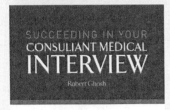

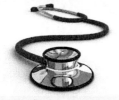

January 2009

240 pages

Paperback

ISBN 978-0-9556746-5-5

£39.99

Achieving Consultant status remains the ambition and pinnacle in the eyes of most hospital doctors. The stakes are high, the competition is intense, and the selection process is discerning. It is important, therefore, that the interview process is understood, and that the commonly asked questions and pitfalls are examined in order to prepare meticulously. Despite the importance of this interview, it is probable that most doctors do not invest sufficient time and effort preparing for it. In this book, the following issues are taken into account:

- Recommendations with regard to preparation prior to application

- Visiting the institution post shortlist-ing, the makeup of the interview panel and presentations

- Behaviour traits to adopt and avoid during the interview

- General principles for answers to commonly asked questions pertain-ing to factual knowledge, opinion and scenarios

- A great portion of the book contains summaries of 'hot topics' with related questions, such as Primary Care Trusts, Foundation Trusts, Govern-ment targets, complaints and risk

The information and guidance given in this book will hopefully go a long way towards helping you with your interview preparation, equipping you with the right behavioural skills and empowering you with the knowledge and confidence to succeed in your Consultant interview.

develop
m e d i c a

More Titles in the Progressing Your Medical Career Series

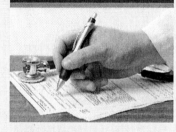

Situational Judgment Tests (SJTs) or Professional Dilemmas form a significant part of the GPST recruitment process and yet many doctors will not have experienced questions of this type under examination conditions. It is therefore essential that candidates sitting the GPST Stage 2 exam have a clear understanding of how to approach questions of this type as poor performance in this section will almost certainly result in not progressing to the Stage 3 selection day.

This interactive book, which contains detailed guidance, and over 70 practice questions (including detailed explanations of all the answers), aims to help doctors prepare for and successfully complete their GPST Stage 2 exam. In this book, Nicole Corriette and Matt Green:

- Describe the context of Situational Judgement Tests within the GPST Stage 2 selection process

- Explore the various ethical principles that you must consider when answering these types of questions

- Set out how to approach the various question types you will be faced with

- Provide over 70 questions to put into practise everything that you learn

- Detailed explanations of the correct answers are also provided to aid your preparations

This engaging, easy to use and comprehensive book is essential reading for anyone serious about excelling in their GPST Stage 2 examination and successfully progressing to Stage 3 of the GPST selection process.

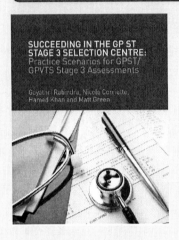

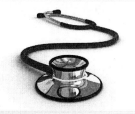

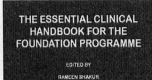
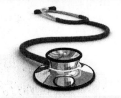